The healing power of
AMINO ACIDS

Clearly written and useful book. — *Natural Food Trader*

By the same author

ACUPUNCTURE TREATMENT OF PAIN
AMINO ACIDS IN THERAPY
BEAT FATIGUE WORKBOOK
CANDIDA ALBICANS
INSTANT PAIN CONTROL
SOFT-TISSUE MANIPULATION
NEW SELF-HELP SERIES:
   ARTHRITIS
   ASTHMA AND HAY FEVER
   HEADACHES AND MIGRAINE
   HIGH BLOOD PRESSURE
   PROSTATE TROUBLES
   SKIN TROUBLES
   VARICOSE VEINS
NEW SLIMMING AND HEALTH WORKBOOK
OSTEOPATHIC SELF-TREATMENT
PROBIOTICS
RADIATION PROTECTION PLAN
YOUR COMPLETE STRESS-PROOFING PROGRAMME

The healing power of AMINO ACIDS

How to boost your health with these amazing new supplements

LEON CHAITOW N.D., D.O.

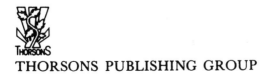

THORSONS PUBLISHING GROUP

First published 1989

This book is dedicated to Don Tyson Ph.D. who is doing so much to allow amino acid therapy to achieve its potential

British Library Cataloguing in Publication Data

Chaitow, Leon
    The healing power of amino acids.
    1. Medicine. Drug therapy. Amino acids
    I. Title
    615'.3137

    ISBN 0-7225-1551-0

Published by Thorsons Publishers Limited, Wellingborough, Northamptonshire, NN8 2RQ, England

Printed in Great Britain by Mackays of Chatham PLC, Chatham, Kent

10 9 8 7 6 5 4 3

Note to readers

Before following the self-help advice given in this book readers are urged to give careful consideration to the nature of their particular health problem, and to consult a competent physician if in any doubt. This book should not be regarded as a substitute for professional medical treatment, and whilst every care is taken to ensure the accuracy of the content, the author and the publishers cannot accept legal responsibility for any problem arising out of the experimentation with the methods described.

In particular, you should ensure that amino acids are purchased from a reputable manufacturer, as many instances have been found of as little as 15 per cent of the labelled material being present in the packaged amino acid supplements. The manufacturers and suppliers listed on page 121 are recommended because they are known to be reliable. This does not mean that the others are unreliable, simply that the author has not had the opportunity to investigate all possible sources.

CONTENTS

INTRODUCTION

Over the next few years we shall all become familiar with some very strange-sounding substances. Ornithine and phenylalanine will trip from our tongues just as we now speak so easily about vitamin C, sodium and potassium.

The 20 amino acids, from which we are made, have been increasingly researched for their amazing healing potential, and for the ability of some of them to powerfully modify mood and behaviour through their influence on the brain and nervous system. This book draws on this research in order to illustrate the power and potential of these amazing amino acids.

The first two chapters give a general account of the ways in which amino acids are acquired by and used in the body. Chapter 3 summarizes the main features of those amino acids which are of most interest in healing (as far as current research goes, that is, for much, much more will be uncovered in years to come). In Chapter 4, I draw on research studies to illustrate briefly the ways in which amino acids (and other nutrient co-factors) have been utilized to encourage healing or to modify behaviour (stopping addictions to alcohol, reducing craving for sugar, modifying violent behaviour, to name some examples). I have not aimed to provide an exhaustive or definitive list of conditions, nor have all the studies been described, by any means. It does however provide a more than adequate introduction to the health-giving potential of amino acid therapy, which should encourage those concerned with the health of their families or themselves to begin to take an interest in these protein fractions which have so much to offer.

The 21st century will undoubtedly see the widespread use of amino acids in therapy and in the prevention of illness. However, it is hoped that those currently involved in advising on nutrition will become aware of the potential of amino acids and that analysis and profiles showing current status will become increasingly available, and hopefully cheaper. This book is dedicated to one pioneer of this new field of nutritional medicine.

1 AMINO ACID THERAPY EXPLAINED

In their search for safe therapeutic substances scientists have recently turned to the 20 or so tiny fractions which make up protein, the amino acids. Here they have found some which have amazing healing powers and which have the ability to alter safely many aspects of the body's functioning. For example, two amino acids, tryptophan and phenylalanine, are some of the most amazingly versatile nutrients which we consume. In fact, they are absolutely vital for life itself! Tryptophan is a natural sleep enhancer, a most effective tranquillizer (in certain circumstances), a safe pain killer, and a useful appetite modifier. Phenylalanine is a potent pain reliever (in one of its two basic forms), a modifier of appetite, and an antidepressant. In all of these roles the way in which either of these substances is taken supplementally, and their occasional combination with other nutrients, are important in ensuring the achievement of satisfactory therapeutic results.

All of these effects and functions result from the biochemical activity of these fractions of protein and with very few exceptions which will be explained, they are completely safe for personal supplementation. *Unlike so many drugs, which can achieve similar results, they are relatively harmless substances which are a normal part of the economy of the body; which the body is used to processing and dealing with every single day; which, when used in a precise manner, can assist in healing a wide variety of health problems.*

Since they are almost always safe, amino acids lend themselves to self-prescription in appropriate conditions which will be outlined.

Meeting a deficiency or pharmacological action?

In therapy which uses nutrients such as vitamins or amino acids there are two possible mechanisms involved. The supplement is either having an actual pharmacological effect, or it may be making good a deficiency which was creating, or aggravating, the condition being treated.

In the first case we are therefore using the substance, be it vitamin C, calcium or an amino acid such as tryptophan, in order to create a biochemical change which will help the body or alter the symptoms. Wherever nutrients are used in this manner there should be a basic understanding of the fact that unless underlying causes of health problems are also being dealt with, the use of a substance, no matter how safe, in order to merely treat symptoms, is probably only a short-term approach.

As an example let us consider a painful condition. If phenylalanine were used to control pain then it is highly likely that the pain would be significantly eased or would disappear entirely. The fascinating pharmacologically induced biochemical events which allow this to happen will be explained in due course. This easing of pain may satisfy the desire to be relieved of unpleasant symptoms, but would it be good for the body, and safe for the individual involved?

The answer must be – not always. Pain is a symptom which warns of underlying problems which require attention, and if the pain is merely suppressed, the ongoing problem would continue and the results could be disastrous. For example, if appendix pain is suppressed it does not stop the appendix from ultimately bursting, with possibly fatal consequences; if an arthritic joint pain is suppressed it does not alter the damaged joint surface, which would become increasingly irritated with the additional use made possible by relief from the warning pain.

Moving away from the example of pain, let us look at another common symptom which can be treated efficiently, but without regard for its causes. If tryptophan is used to induce easy sleep, where insomnia is the result of a hectic lifestyle, poor nutrition or emotional disturbance, without anything being done about the root cause, then improvement would be only short-term. Again, if phenylalanine or tryptophan is used to treat depression, without anything being done to ascertain the causes, be they aspects of lifestyle, diet, emotional problems etc, then again the best interests of the patient would not be served, and almost certainly additional problems would arise in time.

If tryptophan or phenylalanine is used to alter the way we choose our food or the amount we eat (as they both can be) by sending appropriate messages to the brain, we would probably lose weight as desired. However, if the causes of overweight are other than a simple poor choice of food, then the basic problem would remain unaddressed.

All of these examples show how vital it is that causes are dealt with, and not just symptoms. However, there is no reason why symptoms which are bothersome and incapacitating, be they pain, insomnia, depression, excess weight or anything else, should not be treated symptomatically as long as causes are also considered and dealt with.

This theme will be repeated throughout the book, and possible alternative courses of action discussed that might be used as well as these helpful substances and the many other amino acids which we shall be examining.

What about medication and treatment of disease?

Since it is agreed that causes are paramount, and that symptomatic treatment is only part of the way in which we should deal with health problems, it is worth re-emphasizing the difference between the use of these natural substances and drugs, which also attack symptoms.

Drugs are seldom, with very few exceptions, natural parts of the economy of the body. When aspirin, for example, is given for pain control it causes a variety of chemical changes to occur, some of which are desirable in that pain is relieved, while others are undesirable in that they actually harm the body. This is true of ALL drugs, without exception: there is no such thing as a completely safe drug. They all work by altering normal body processes, sometimes with severely undesirable complications. When we speak of a substance altering the body processes, in any way, we refer to the pharmacological use of that substance.

Broadly speaking, pain-killing drugs are divided into the steroid drugs and the non-steroid, anti-inflammatory (known as NSAIDS, which stands for Non-steroid Anti-inflammatory Drugs) and other forms of pain killing drugs. All of these have produced fatalities and serious health problems in their wake, and many have been withdrawn from general use because of these side-effects. Others continue to be used since the therapeutic advantages produced, in terms of symptoms controlled, seems to doctors, in many cases, to outweigh the potential dangers. Phenylalanine, on the other hand, acts in a completely different manner as a pain relieving agent. Rather than 'killing' pain this substance merely slows down the normal breakdown, in the body, of naturally occurring pain killers (endorphins etc) produced by the body itself, and so the beneficial effects achieved are not 'bought' at any cost to the overall health of the person involved. This will be explained in greater detail in later sections. At this point it is only necessary to have an appreciation of the fact that amino acids are (with a few specific exceptions which will be explained) safe, and not potentially dangerous in the way drugs are, even when they are being used pharmacologically.

Amino acids when used as described in this book do not involve toxic substances. They are fractions of the normal protein foods we eat every day. Amino acids are part of our daily lives, and by selectively ingesting a greater concentration of one or other, or a combination, of these, at appropriate times, we can safely help relieve many undesirable symptoms, while hopefully at the same time paying attention to the reasons for the problem.

Deficiency

When we take amino acid supplements we may often be making good a deficiency of the substance, or be correcting the balance between a number of nutrients, and in this way we may be helping to relieve symptoms. In this case, the action produced by the supplementation is not pharmacological, but rather a replenishing of a needed substance.

One thing is certain in medicine, drugs are not a natural part of the economy of the body and therefore can never be replacements for deficient substances. The body is never deficient in aspirin, for example, although it may well be deficient in an amino acid, or have an imbalanced ratio between a number of these, or between other essential nutrients, due to amino acid deficiency or imbalance.

We have become used to the concept of using certain nutrient substances in a therapeutic or preventative manner. For example, vitamin C is commonly used for its beneficial effect in infections such as influenza; B complex vitamins are commonly used to help in a variety of nerve problems; calcium is used to assist in replenishment of bone when there exists decalcification (osteoporosis for example), or for its prevention. Amino acids are nutrient substances, just as minerals and vitamins are, and have at least as large a range of beneficial characteristics.

Why we may sometimes be 'short' of amino acids

It is legitimate to ask the question, 'why should we ever be short of adequate amino acids, considering the amounts of protein consumed?' The answer is not a simple one but requires that we examine a number of factors which can interact to produce deficiency in the midst of plenty. Professor Jeffrey Bland has coined the phrase 'the undernutrition of overconsumption', and this is to an extent a factor. In contrast to many underdeveloped countries where malnutrition is the result of underconsumption, not enough to eat, in many industrialized countries a different form of malnutrition, caused by overeating, exists. More specifically it arises partly as a result of eating devitalized, over-refined and adulterated foods, and partly as a result of a number of conditions which mitigate against adequate digestion of what is eaten.

In order to be utilized by the body the amino acids derived from food have to be in what is termed their 'free' form. In other words, they need to be 'unlocked' from the chains of protein in which form they exist in our food and are consumed. In protein, as it is eaten in the form of eggs, meat, nuts etc., the 20 amino acids are present in the particular ratios characteristic of that food or substance, and it is in the digestive process that these are broken down into their individual components, for absorption by the body and ultimate resynthesis in the system to build new cells, tissues and organs. If, for whatever reason, this breakdown into units of free amino acids does not occur, then the body cannot build up the new tissues it needs for health and efficiency. Thus, in an ocean of protein being consumed, there may be too little of the very substances of which protein is made, the individual amino acids.

'Water, water everywhere, yet not a drop to drink'. Thus spoke the Ancient Mariner who, surrounded by salt water, could not find a drinkable drop. Modern man with his vast intake of protein-rich dairy foods and meat products is often in the same position in relation to the amino acids upon which his body and life depend.

Why? The digestive factor

One of the reasons for this is the often inadequate quantity or efficiency of the digestive juices produced in the stomach and pancreas, when the pancreas fails to produce essential protein digesting enzymes. Excessive demands upon any organ in the body can in time lead to its abilities becoming exhausted.

The pancreas produces the so called proteolytic enzymes, such as trypsin, chymotrypsin etc, for protein digestion. It also has the major task of producing insulin with which the body attempts to control sugar levels in the bloodstream. When this particular function breaks down diabetes occurs. Diabetes is all too common in modern society, and is related directly to overconsumption of fats and sugars. If proteolytic enzyme production by the pancreas is inadequate then amino acid breakdown is faulty, and as a result the body will have a serious lack of the raw materials from which to make more enzymes, and so the cycle repeats itself and worsens with time. Poor digestion leads to poor amino acid breakdown, which leads to worse digestion.

Other substances which harm the pancreas, apart from sugar and fats, are alcohol, coffee, cigarettes and a number of drugs. Apart from aberrant insulin production, other symptoms which might become apparent when pancreatic function is impaired are recurrent gastritis and frequent allergic type reactions, related to incompletely digested substances being absorbed into the bloodstream.

If at the same time protein intake is high, there are even greater demands being made on a compromised digestive system with the pancreas labouring even harder, in vain, to produce substances it is unable to produce.

Other digestive imbalances, including the all too common in-adequacy of the gastric secretions of hydrochloric acid or pepsin, can result in similar incomplete digestion of proteins, and therefore in poor free amino acid presence in the 'pool' of amino acids from which the body draws the raw materials with which to reconstruct and constantly renew itself.

The allergic factor

The whole process of incomplete digestion is a key to understand-ing many allergic problems. These may result from partially digested substances (and toxic debris associated with bacteria which interact with them) crossing into the bloodstream and causing reactions with the immune (defence) system of the body. A wide range of physical and mental symptoms can often then result.

Summary of protein digestion

In brief, the pattern of digestion by which the body is supplied with adequate amino acids in their free form (no longer still in chains) is as follows.

Entering the mouth in large chunks, protein needs to be chew-ed sufficiently to reduce the portions to fragments so that the sur-faces of these portions are accessible to the digestive juices. If chewing is poor, then the protein is less likely to be broken down into its constituents later on in the digestive process. In the stomach a variety of juices, such as hydrochloric acid and pepsin (an enzyme), work on the protein, and about 15 per cent of it should be digested by the time the food moves on to the small intestine.

As we have noted above, if hydrochloric acid or the proteolytic enzymes are in short supply even this modest amount of digestion will be absent. It is a fact that as we grow older so our production of hydrochloric acid decreases, and it is estimated that by the age of 60 fully a third of individuals no longer secrete any stomach acids at all. The protein intake of such people may be prodigious but their actual absorption will be very limited.

Having reached the small intestine it is vital that a correct degree of local acidity be present so that specific enzymes can un-couple the amino acids from each other. If the acidity is incorrect because of digestive problems, or if the enzymes required to 'un-hook' the amino acids are deficient, then only partially digested proteins will be left.

This will lead to bowel putrefaction, and a great deal of gas will be formed and toxic substances (by-products of this putrefaction induced by bowel bacteria on the partially digested protein) will be absorbed into the bloodstream.

If, however, the digestive juices are working well, on well chewed protein, and the residue reaches the small intestine to be worked on by a plentiful supply of the correct enzymes which then unhook the individual amino acids into their free form, these are then absorbed into the bloodstream where they form a pool of reserve material for use in the sound construction of new body tissues and substances, either on their own or in combination with factors such as minerals and/or vitamins.

From the above it should be quite clear that we cannot ensure the presence of amino acids in the body simply by eating ade-quate protein. Whatever the reasons for the inadequate digestion of protein, it is obvious that there can be an actual deficiency in certain amino acids due to one of the following factors:

• a poor diet.
• incomplete breakdown of proteins in the digestive system.
• inherited abnormalities in the biochemical mechanisms of the body.

In addition, there is also the factor of biochemical individuality.

Biochemical individuality

This term refers to our own particular idiosyncratic needs for cer-tain nutrients, which are now established scientifically. Thus one person may require five to seven times as much calcium or vitamin C as another in order to remain in good health, while another person may require three or four times as much vitamin A and/or zinc. We are told that we require certain levels of nutrient intake to maintain health. These figures (RDAs, for recommended daily allowances) relate to averages and, thus far, in extensive testing, very few people have been found who fit the average for ALL nutrients.

Professor Roger Williams of Texas University has declared that we all have unique biochemical requirements, which relate both to acquired and to inherited factors.

This means that for each of us, the quantity of each nutrient in our diet is different. Indeed, from the range of almost 50 substances which should be present in our diet (vitamins, minerals, trace elements, amino acids, essential fatty acids etc.) and which are essential for life, there are requirements which are different for each of us. And so we each need different amounts of amino acids, just as we need different amounts of vitamins, minerals, essential fatty acids or trace elements.

How we can measure amino acid imbalances

It is possible to study amino acid levels and ratios (the relationship of amino acids to each other in quantitative terms) by analysing urine, serum and other tissues. Such amino acid 'profiles' have shown definite patterns which relate to different conditions, so that it is now possible to give certain amino acids as supplements for various chronic diseases and general health problems. This is being done with great effect in cases of AIDS and chronic fungal infections such as Candida albicans. Thus amino acids can be used to supplement deficiencies, by giving one or other of these as a means of restoring normal levels or ratios, and therefore normal function.

In these cases, although part of the real cause of the problem is being taken care of, the reasons why deficiency of the substance exists still needs to be ascertained and dealt with, if possible (it may sometimes relate to genetic abnormalities which cannot be corrected). In other cases, as discussed earlier, amino acids are prescribed in order to achieve a pharmacological effect, there being no evidence of amino acid deficiency. Here the cause of the problem is not being addressed and without this happening real health, as opposed to relief of symptoms, cannot be regained.

We shall now pass on to look at the nature and composition of amino acids.

2 ABOUT AMINO ACIDS

Amino acids can best be described as the construction blocks from which protein is made. Just as in a child's construction kit the pieces come in different shapes and sizes and yet fit together to make something recognizable, so the more than 20 amino acids each have unique characteristics, and yet are capable of being fitted together into an almost limitless variety of proteins.

Protein is formed by the joining together, into chains, of amino acids and thus far over 100,000 different proteins have been identified in nature, which are the result of variations in the pattern in which the chains are constructed.

The human body alone contains over 50,000 different forms of protein. The total presence of amino acids in the body represents fully three quarters of the body's dry weight (this is excluding the water content). Most of the amino acids in the body can be manufactured out of just eight other amino acids, which are all essential in the diet. This means that our diet has to allow the acquisition of free forms of these eight amino acids for life to continue.

These 'essential' amino acids are critically important to life and health, for out of them the body makes the other amino acids, as well as many of the vital compounds which keep the body working, such as the enzymes, neurotransmitters, mucopolysaccharides etc., not to mention blood, muscles, organs and bones from which we are constructed.

When only a short chain of amino acids is joined together, in a particular sequence, it is called a peptide. When the chain is long, it is called a protein.

The amino acids themselves are constructed from a combination of the following elements: carbon, hydrogen, oxygen, nitrogen and in some cases sulphur.

Every amino acid comes in two forms, a 'left-handed' (L) and a 'right-handed' (D) form. These two forms are identical in every respect except for the conformation of the sub-units of which they are composed. That is to say, although chemically they contain the same elements, in precisely the same quantities and in the same sequence, they are the mirror image of each other, just as the human left hand has the same construction as the human right hand and yet they are different (a right hand cannot wear a left-handed glove for example). Protein chains cannot be formed from a combination of L and D amino acids.

The body is constructed almost without exception from the L forms of amino acid. However, the D forms, which occur in nature, are often found to have therapeutic value and, as we shall see later, the D form of phenylalanine is a particularly valuable asset in treating pain.

The essential amino acids which are required by the adult body (children have slightly different needs, as we shall see) to make the other amino acids as well as the proteins of the body are: L–tryptophan, L–isoleucine, L–lysine, L–threonine, L–leucine, L–methionine, L–phenylalanine, L–valine. Henceforth, we shall drop the 'L' prefix so that it can always be assumed that a named amino acid is the L form. D forms, or a combination of D and L forms, will be clearly described as such. From these raw materials, which are essential elements in the diet, the body synthesizes the other amino acids (non-essential) which are *cysteine, cystine, tyrosine, arginine, alanine, glutamic acid, proline, hydroxyproline, glutamine, histidine, aspartic acid, glycine, serine, asparginine, carnitine.*

Recent research, however, has questioned the concept of essential and non-essential amino acids. Arginine for example is known to be in short supply in children, and may therefore be considered 'essential' for them, because the young body is incapable of manufacturing adequate amounts from the other essential raw materials, as an adult body can. Histidine is also considered necessary in the diet of infants, whereas it is not considered by all experts to be an essential amino acid for adults.

Furthermore, it is now known that, under certain conditions, any amino acid can become essential. Such a situation may arise when demand for it is increased under certain conditions of stress (intense heat or cold, shock etc) or illness (fever) or during pregnancy, for example. Drugs or toxic factors can also put undue strain on the normal levels of particular amino acids, which would transfer them from a non-essential to an essential status. There are also a variety of inherited anomalies which can lead to deficiencies, and/or excesses, of amino acids in the body. The so-called branch-chain amino acids (leucine, isoleucine, valine) account for the bulk of such problems.

Professor Jeffrey Bland, a noted American researcher into nutrition, calls normally non-essential amino acids, which become essential, 'contingent', and describes histidine in this way, especially in allergic situations where large amounts of the substance histamine, which derives from the amino acid histidine, is utilized by the body.

Under certain specific conditions all amino acids are therefore potentially essential for bodily health to be maintained.

Amino acids in digestion

As we have seen in Chapter 1, presence of a substance in the diet is not of itself enough, for until the amino acid, locked into the food, is broken down by digestion into its single free form, the body cannot use it. Thus, *simply telling a person to eat foods containing the amino acid which is required is not enough.* Free form acids must be provided in supplement form, in order to ensure therapeutic results. Some common proteins are rich in certain amino acids and poor in others. The least well supplied amino acid in any particular food is called the 'limiting' amino acid.

Amino acids do not work in isolation, but are dependent upon vitamins and minerals in order to form body tissues such as bone and muscle, hormones and enzymes. For example, the amino acid tyrosine needs to combine with iodine for the thyroid hormone thyroxin to be created: thyroxin cannot be manufactured without both these substances.

The over-emphasis of nutritionists on the importance to health of vitamins and minerals has distracted attention from the amino acids. As already mentioned, this is largely because of the widespread assumption that if there was enough protein in the diet then we would automatically get all the amino acids we needed. However the body requires daily at least 20 times as much in amino acid intake as it does in vitamins, and about four times as much as the minerals. This requirement has to be in the form of free amino acids to be of any value, not protein in undigested lumps. It is only when we have an efficient digestive function that such a breakdown of protein can occur, releasing an adequate supply of free amino acids.

In good health, the body is constantly breaking down many of its own constituent cells for recycling, as well as ingested protein from food. Both of these tasks require the presence of specific enzymes in order to uncouple the amino acids from the chains into which they are linked as proteins. If a particular enzyme is deficient, then this uncoupling task is not properly accomplished and free amino acid deficiency will occur, causing in turn further enzyme deficiency, and even poorer subsequent protein breakdown.

The other functions of amino acids

Amino acids also play a vital role in a number of body processes such as the urea cycle, the complex process whereby ammonia is detoxified from the body. Ammonia is a constant product of muscle metabolism and nitrogen use in the body, and we would die were it not metabolized adequately. Amino acids achieve this, arginine and ornithine being mainly involved.

Another body cycle called the citric acid cycle (or Krebs cycle) is related to the expiration of carbon dioxide and hydrogen, and the potential for production of energy, and for counteracting excessive acidity, via a complex interaction of amino acids and other substances. The complexities of the interactions between the citric acid cycle and the urea cycle, and manifold dangers caused by faults in these systems, are beyond the scope of this book. However, they are worth a mention in order to further emphasize the importance of amino acids, which are crucial in these life preserving functions of detoxification and energy production.

Apart from being the primary construction material for tissue, bone, organs, hormones, neurotransmitters, enzymes etc., amino acids are the raw material from which the genetic coding material of every cell in the body, DNA, is constructed. They are also a vital part of the immune system, the body's defence mechanism.

Amino acids and neurotransmitters

Individual types of amino acids have particular characteristics. Some are capable of influencing body processes because they are essential to the formation of neurotransmitters, substances which are used in the brain and by the nervous system to increase or decrease the efficiency and rapidity of nerve transmission. The ability of the brain to receive and to transmit messages depends upon these neurotransmitters, which are themselves dependent upon particular amino acids. All functions of the body depend upon sound nervous interconnection. This allows organs and muscles to report back to the higher centres as to their status, and for receiving instructions from the higher centres, as to their behaviour and needs. The coordination and regulation of all the millions of messages that are constantly going on in the body, depend upon neurotransmitters and therefore on amino acids. Amino acids are especially important where nerves interact (synapse), where information is passed on and received. Some of the neurotransmitters have a stimulating, excitatory function and others have a calming, inhibitory function.

The scope and use of appropriate amino acids in therapy can therefore be seen to be enormous. Unless all the amino acids, in their free form, are present in adequate amounts, there will be imbalances in the neurotransmitter function, and a variety of nervous and emotional problems will result. The very energy of the brain is dependent upon certain amino acids. The two amino acids used as examples of the value of this class of nutrients in Chapter 1, tryptophan and phenylalanine, are both of profound importance in their relation to brain and nerve function, as we shall see.

Another major area of activity of some of the amino acids is as detoxifiers of the body. The sulphur rich amino acids (methionine, cysteine, cystine) are especially capable of this sometimes life-saving task. These have the ability to chelate (lock onto) heavy metals such as lead, mercury and aluminium, which are toxic to the body, and to actually remove them from the system.

They are also capable of damping down damaging processes in the body relating to oxidation of certain substances such as fats. When toxic substances are present in tissue or in the bloodstream, there is potential for what is called free radical damage, as fractions of the oxidizing substance cascade around the area creating tissue damage. These processes which are thought to result in such cell changes as occur in arteries before they become atherosclerotic, and to cells before they become cancerous, are controlled by free radical scavengers or quenchers, of which the sulphur rich amino acids are a major part. Vitamins A, C, and E and the mineral selenium are also antioxidants which reduce free radical damage.

In the next chapters we shall look at the roles which have been defined for the amino acids as well as their major therapeutic effects.

Future research will doubtless open up new avenues of therapeutic potential, as it will also most certainly discover new amino acids. Several of these have been noted in the past few years such as γ-carboxyglutamic acid and β-carboxyaspartic acid. What we have at present is a working knowledge of the major amino acids, with a fair idea of how to use these therapeutically. Protein power is now available for us to use in the quest for better health.

3 AMINO ACIDS: SUMMARY OF FUNCTIONS AND THERAPEUTIC USES

This chapter looks in detail at those free form amino acids which can be safely used for supplementation. The ways in which these have been, and can be, utilized is described more fully in Chapter 4, which looks at individual health complaints, and in which research evidence as to the benefits derived from use of amino acids is presented, as is information about dosage.

Before using an amino acid therapeutically read about its usefulness in Chapter 4, and also refer to the notes given in the chapter about its many different characteristics. This will give you an understanding of the substance and alert you to possible problems (e.g. clashes with other medicines) and also details of how to enhance its effectiveness by combining it with other nutrients and methods (best taken with vitamin C, or with another amino acid etc).

When to take an amino acid, or a combination of them, is also a key element in its effectiveness. With very few exceptions, which are discussed in the text, this should always be away from mealtimes, otherwise amino acids will be competing for absorption with the proteins present in the food of the meal. Free form amino acids are readily and speedily absorbed when taken an hour before or an hour and a half after a meal, with plain water.

Not all of the many functions of amino acids which go to make up, and which are at work in, the body, have as yet been clearly identified, and by no means all of the therapeutic uses have as yet been discovered. The following summary of the characteristics, functions and uses of amino acids is not exhaustive, since some amino acids have been ascribed only minor roles thus far.

Just as we have come to be aware of the nutrient content of food in terms of vitamins and minerals (oranges and lemons for vitamin C etc), so in time we shall become familiar with amino acids and their different balances found in certain foods. For instance, already those people following a high lysine/low arginine diet for conditions such as herpes are able to select their foods (no chocolate, low intake of nuts and wholegrains, high intake of fruits, fish and chicken etc) appropriately. Hopefully in time this will become second nature to those of us whose unique biochemical requirements demand that to be healthy a particular balance of amino acids is best. This will include a great many people.

Supplementation will be seen to be a logical and safe approach to achieving good health (as long as basic care is taken over factors such as their occasional undesirable combination with certain other substances, and the ways they should be used in certain conditions, all of which are listed in various places in the book).

Use this book as a guide to where these marvellous protein fractions can help you, by discovering their power and understanding their potential.

Arginine

- An essential amino acid for children but not for adults.
- Secreted by the anterior pituitary gland.
- Stimulates human growth hormone (HGH) which stimulates immune (defence) function.
- Accelerates wound healing.
- Plays major part in urea cycle which detoxifies ammonia from the system (in this cycle it is converted to ornithine and then back to arginine).
- Necessary for normal sperm count.
- Involved in glucose (sugar) control mechanisms in the blood (Glucose Tolerance Factor).
- Enhances fat metabolism.
- Involved in insulin production.

Therapeutic uses
- Benefits to arthritics.
- Inhibition of tumour development.
- Helpful in some forms of infertility.
- Stimulates production of T-cells (major part of immune system) and enhances wound and burn healing.

Deficiency
- Infertility in males.
- Premature ageing.
- Toxicity and increase in free radical activity.
- Overweight.

Excess
- Enhanced virus replication (eg herpes simplex) unless adequate lysine also present.
- Aggravation of certain forms of schizophrenia.

Genetically acquired disorder
- Hyperargininaemia, which can be satisfactorily treated medically.

Caution
- Schizophrenics should use with caution.
- Avoid with herpes.

Aspartic acid

- Has protective functions for the liver and assists in detoxification of ammonia.
- Promotes uptake of trace elements in the gut and is involved in the energy cycle.
- Acts to transport magnesium and potassium to cells and is part of the sweetener aspartame (together with phenylalanine).

Therapeutic use
- Pronounced relief of fatigue has been noted in three quarters of patients supplemented with potassium and magnesium aspartate (1 g daily) (see page 73).

Histidine

- Is metabolized into the neurotransmitter histamine, which is involved in smooth muscle function, and contraction and dilation (expansion) of blood vessels.
- Is required for sexual arousal.
- Helps maintain the myelin sheaths which insulate the nerves and is required by the auditory nerve for good function.
- Stimulates production of red and white blood cells.
- Two forms of schizophrenia have been noted, which are characterized by either excessive or low levels of histamine in the body (brain).
- Best taken with vitamin C.

Therapeutic uses
- Protects against radiation damage (it was used in the Russian space programme).
- Chelates (helps to remove) toxic metals from the body.
- Has been successfully used in the treatment of rheumatoid arthritis.
- Useful together with vitamins B3 and B6 in normalizing problems of poor sexual arousal.
- Effective in treating ulcers in the digestive tract.
- Effective in treating nausea during pregnancy.

Deficiency
- Leads to poor hearing or deafness.

Genetically acquired disorder
- Histidineaemia, which can be satisfactorily treated medically.

Caution
- Should be used cautiously by manic depressive patients who have elevated levels of histamine (see page 113).
- Women with severe premenstrual depression should avoid histidine supplementation.

Leucine and isoleucine

- Essential amino acids.
- Together with valine, they comprise the group of amino acids known as branched chain amino acids.
- They should always be supplemented in combination with

each other unless a particular strategy is being adopted therapeutically.

- Both are commonly deficient in amino acid profiles of chronically sick individuals.
- Isoleucine is useful in formation of haemoglobin.

Therapeutic uses
- Leucine is useful in Parkinson's disease.
- D-leucine may be effective as enhancer of pain killing effects of naturally produced endorphins (as is phenylalanine).

Deficiency
- Common in cases of chronic physical and mental disease.

Excess
- May predispose to pellagra.

Valine

- An essential amino acid which is needed for normalizing the nitrogen balance in the body.
- The third (together with leucine and isoleucine) of the group known as branched chain amino acids.
- Vital for mental function, muscle coordination and neural function.

Therapeutic uses
- Helpful in cases of inflammation.

Excess
- Sensations of 'crawling skin' and hallucinations.

Deficiency
- Nervousness.
- Poor sleep patterns and mental symptoms.
- Negative nitrogen balance (toxicity).

Genetically acquired disorders
- Hypervalinaemia.
- Methylmalonic aciduria.
- MSUD (maple syrup urine disease). Presents in newborn babies with vomiting, lethargy, tight muscles, fits and unless treated correctly, death follows very shortly afterwards. Some forms begin later in life. A special diet low in the branch-

chained amino acids is needed and in some forms of the disease, the vitamin thiamin (B1) is also helpful.

Lysine

- An essential amino acid often low in vegetarian diets.
- Important for children's growth and development.
- Involved in synthesis of the amino acid carnitine (see below), therefore important in fat metabolism.
- Helps in the formation of antibodies to fight disease.

Therapeutic uses
- Has been shown to be effective in treatment of herpes simplex virus, especially when combined with vitamin C and a low arginine diet. This pattern is also thought to decrease chances of atherosclerotic changes (see pages 52 and 77.)
- Enhances concentration.

Deficiency
- Fatigue, dizziness, anaemia, visual disorders, nausea.
- Dietary deficiency of lysine leads to increased calcium excretion and therefore higher danger of kidney stones.

Genetically acquired disorder
- Hyperlysinaemia, which can be satisfactorily treated medically.

Phenylalanine

- An essential amino acid.
- The precursor (parent substance) of tyrosine and hence of dopamine, norepinephrine (noradrenaline) and epinephrine (adrenaline) for which vitamins B6 and C are required in the biochemical conversion processes. These substances control or affect heart rate and output, blood pressure, oxygen consumption, blood sugar levels, fat metabolism and many functions of the brain.
- Cannot be metabolized without adequate vitamin C.
- Required by the thyroid for normal function.

Therapeutic uses
L-phenylalanine
- Stimulates production of cholescystokinin, inducing satiety

(feeling of having eaten enough). It is therefore useful in weight control.
- Acts as an antidepressant.

D-phenylalanine
- Powerful non-toxic, non-addictive enhancer of endogenous (produced by the body itself) pain killers (by slowing down their normal degradation).
- Reduces symptoms of multiple sclerosis and Parkinson's disease.
- Acts as an antidepressant.
- May improve memory, concentration and mental alertness.

D-L phenylalanine
- Pain control.
- Antidepressant.
- Treats symptoms of rheumatoid arthritis.
- Treats the depigmentation occurring in the skin condition vitiligo (together with ultra violet light).

Deficiency
- In childhood, leads to tyrosine deficiency and therefore mental retardation, as well as melanin deficiency which makes eczema more likely.
- In adults, leads to emotional disorders, weight gain, circulatory problems.

Genetically acquired disorders
- Hyperphenylalanineaemias which include phenylketonuria (PKU), a common amino acidopathy (affecting one in 14,000 babies in North America). PKU leads to mental retardation and lack of pigmentation. This is treated by diets low in phenylalanine. Rapid detection is essential if prevention of the worse symptoms is to be effective.

Dangers of phenylalanine
- Should not be used by anyone currently taking any of the monoamine oxidase inhibitor drugs (MAO).
- Should be used with caution by anyone with high blood pressure.
- Should be avoided by phenylketonurics and by pregnant or lactating women.

Tryptophan

- An essential amino acid, needed for synthesis of nicotinic acid (vitamin B3) in the body and the precursor of the neurotransmitter serotonin which is a calming sedating substance essential for normal mood and sleep patterns.
- Influences the amount of protein chosen at meals and is therefore used to control weight reduction.
- Uptake of tryptophan by the brain is enhanced by vitamin B6 and vitamin C.
- Acts as a mood stabilizer (calms agitation, stimulates depressed individuals).
- The less tryptophan the greater the degree of emotional disturbance.

Therapeutic uses
- Useful in some forms of vascular migraine.
- Has anti-depressant potential.
- Useful in weight control.
- A powerful sleep enhancer when combined with magnesium and vitamin B6.
- Menopausal depressive conditions.
- Has powerful pain killing effects.
- Useful for individuals with Parkinson's disease who are taking levo-dopa drugs.
- Helps symptoms of 'restless legs syndrome'.
- May be helpful in treating rheumatoid arthritis (animal studies).
- May help patients with tardive dyskinesia.

Caution
- May be dangerous if used in pregnancy.
- May aggravate bronchial asthma.
- May aggravate the auto-immune condition lupus.

Deficiency
- Insomnia, mental disturbance and depression.
- Poor skin colouring and tone, and brittle fingernails.
- Indigestion.
- Craving for carbohydrate.

Carnitine

- This is synthesized in the liver from lysine and methionine, vitamin C being essential for its conversion.
- Men have greater physiological need for carnitine than women.
- Influences sperm motility; reduces triglyceride levels in the blood and protects the heart against myocardial infarction by removing free fatty acids.
- Has a major role in transferring fatty acids into cells where they are used as energy sources.
- Aids in mobilizing fatty deposits in obesity and helps in removal of ketones (fat waste products) from the blood.

Therapeutic uses
- Useful in treating some forms of infertility.
- Reduces high levels of triglycerides in the blood.
- Reduces surface fats in conditions such as cellulite.
- Helpful in circulatory problems such as intermittent claudication.
- Reduces feelings of fatigue and muscle weakness.
- Helpful in treatment of fatty liver degeneration and alcohol damage to liver.
- May be useful (with other nutrients) in helping glucose tolerance in diabetics.
- Also used in cardiac disease (especially myocardial ischemia – lack of oxygen reaching heart muscle); muscular dystrophy and other myopathies and neuromuscular diseases; obesity.

Dangers and side effects
- Two thirds of patients treated using carnitine report gastrointestinal side effects or increased body odour which disappeared or diminished with continued use at a lower dosage.
- Especial care should be taken in supplementing carnitine to people with kidney damage.

Tyrosine

- Derived from phenylalanine and is a precursor of the thyroid hormones, as well as of dopa, dopamine, norepinephrine

(noradrenaline) and epinephrine (adrenaline).
* Aids in normal brain function and in treating abnormal brain function as a supplier of neurotransmitters.

Therapeutic uses
* Useful in Parkinson's disease and some cases of depression which are not amenable to treatment with tryptophan.
* Small doses of tyrosine are often more effective than large ones in increasing brain neurotransmitter levels.
* Effective in alleviating hay fever and grass allergies.

Glutamic acid and glutamine

* Under certain conditions, these may become essential amino acids.
* They are the dominant amino acids of the cerebro-spinal fluid and serum.
* Glutamine readily passes through the blood/brain barrier (glutamic acid does not).
* Glutamic acid is readily converted from glutamine and is a uniquely powerful 'brain' fuel.
* Glutamic acid gives rise to GABA, a calming agent in the brain and possibly a neurotransmitter.
* Glutamic acid is required for manufacture of the B vitamin folic acid.
* Glutamic acid is a component of the glucose tolerance factor.
* Glutamine is useful in maintaining the body's nitrogen balance.
* Needed for what is called transamination (the production of other non-essential amino acids).

Therapeutic uses
Glutamic acid
* Used in treating childhood behavioural problems.
* Re-converts to glutamine and thus detoxifies the brain from ammonia.
* Has been shown in laboratory studies to dissolve or retard formation of kidney stones.
Glutamine
* Protects the body from the effects of alcohol and decreases the desire for it, and in some cases for sugar.

- Helps heal peptic ulceration (400 mg 4 × daily before meals and before retiring).
- Useful in cases of depression.
- Blunts carbohydrate cravings, therefore helpful in treatment of obesity.
- May help in some cases of schizophrenia and senility.
- Treats fatigue.
- Used to raise IQs and for memory improvement.

Deficiency
- Can lead to cantankerous and grouchy behaviour.

Toxicity
- May result from excessive glutamine intake (over 2 g daily may lead to manic behaviour).

Methionine

- An essential amino acid containing sulphur.
- A power antioxidant preventing free radical damage to tissues.
- Assisted by vitamin B6.
- Helps produce choline and adrenaline, lecithin and vitamin B12.
- Assists gallbladder function through synthesis of bile salts.
- The precursor of the amino acids taurine, cystine and cysteine.
- Acts to detoxify heavy metals from the body and also excessive levels of histamine (which is part of histadelic schizophrenia symptomatology).
- Strengthens hair follicles.
- Detoxifies the liver, preventing buildup of excess fats.
- Essential for selenium bioavailability in the body.

Therapeutic uses
- Helps relieve arthritic and rheumatic symptoms.
- Useful in cases requiring detoxification and antioxidation.
- May retard cataract development.
- Helpful in some cases of Parkinson's disease (1 g daily, rising to 5 g for two months).
- Detoxifies excessive histamine levels found in some forms of schizophrenia.

- May be useful in gallbadder problems relating to oestrogen excess, resulting from contraceptive medication.

Deficiency
- Leads to poor skin tone, hair loss, toxic waste buildup, fatty infiltration of the liver, anaemia, retarded protein synthesis, atherosclerosis.

Genetically acquired disorders
- Hypermethionineaemia for which therapy is not indicated.

Taurine

- This neurotransmitter is manufactured in the body from methionine or cysteine in the liver, and vitamin B6 is needed for its synthesis. One of the sulphur rich group of amino acids, the major supply should come from the diet, where it is only found in foods of animal origin.
- Women require more taurine than men, since female hormone oestradiol is found to inhibit its synthesis in the liver.
- Interacts with bile salts to maintain their solubility, and with cholesterol, preventing gall stones.
- Taurine levels rise in serum as zinc levels decrease, leading to low brain levels of taurine which are undesirable. Zinc is therefore vital to its use.
- The most prevalent amino acid in the heart, it helps conserve potassium and calcium in the heart muscle thereby helping it to function better. Research continues to ascertain its precise role(s) in heart function, which is thought to be profoundly important.
- Influences insulin and blood sugar levels.
- Greater concentrations of taurine are found in the pineal and pituitary glands after exposure to natural full spectrum light. People deprived of this may become mentally impaired and depressed, which may relate to taurine lack.
- Increases in use when the individual is under stress.
- Only found in the L form.
- The second most prevalent amino acid in human milk but is poorly supplied in cow's milk.

Therapeutic uses
- Helpful in some types of epilepsy.
- Cardiac conditions such as congestive heart failure and atherosclerosis, stress and eye problems; compromised immune function.
- Also useful in gallbladder disease.
- Claimed to enhance IQ levels in Down's syndrome children (together with other nutrients).

Deficiency
- In children, may lead to epilepsy.
- In adults, when there is also zinc deficiency, may lead to eye problems.

Cysteine

- Derived from methionine or serine in the liver.
- A major sulphur containing amino acid (together with methionine and taurine).
- A powerful antioxidant.
- Part of tripeptide glutathione (see below) which is itself part of what is known as glucose tolerance factor (GTF) as well as being a major detoxifying agent.
- Should not be confused with cystine which is a similar but not identical substance which does not possess the antioxidant qualities of cysteine.
- Converts to cystine in the absence of adequate vitamin C.
- Cystine and cysteine are vital for adequate use in the body of vitamin B6.
- In chronic disease the formation of methionine into cysteine is often prevented.
- Contributes towards the strength of the hair (over 10 per cent of hair is cysteine) and also in enzyme and insulin production.
- Skin texture and flexibility are related to cysteine function by virtue of free radical inactivation.

Therapeutic uses
- Cysteine can usefully be supplemented in all cases of chronic disease.
- Removes heavy metals from the body, and protects against the effects of alcohol, cigarette smoking and pollution etc, by ensuring detoxification of acetaldehyde.

- Useful in iron deficiency, and is helpful in prevention of cataracts.

Caution
- Cysteine should be used with caution by diabetics.

Cystine

- This is part of insulin molecule.
- One of the sulphur rich amino acid group.
- Acts as a heavy metal chelator.

Therapeutic uses
- Useful in treatment of skin problems such as psoriasis and eczema.
- Helps tissues to heal after surgery.

Caution
- People predisposed to kidney or liver stones should take care in use of cystine.

Glutathione

- A tripeptide made up of the amino acids cysteine, glutamic acid and glycine.
- Inhibits damage to fat cells induced by free radical activity and retards the ageing process.
- Neutralizes dangerous atmospheric substances such as petrocarbons and chlorine.
- Because of its cysteine content it has a sulphur element which accounts for its detoxification potential.

Therapeutic uses
- Has been shown to protect the liver against alcohol induced damage.
- Protects against radiation effects.
- Chelates heavy metals from the system.
- Causes regression of tumours in animals.
- Has been noted to be in short supply in tissues of diabetics where it acts on accumulated dehydroascorbic acid to produce vitamin C.

Gamma-aminobutyric acid (GABA)

- A non-essential amino acid formed from glutamic acid.
- Helps regulate nerve function and enhances the ability of vitamin B3 (niacinamide) to act.

Therapeutic uses
- Induces calmness and tranquillity in cases of manic behaviour, acute agitation, schizophrenia, epilepsy and high blood pressure.
- Helpful in cases of enlarged prostate gland by stimulating the release of the prolactin hormone from the pituitary, resulting in reduction in size.

Glycine

- A non-essential amino acid which is part of the tripeptide glutathione, which is a detoxifying agent, especially for the liver.
- Essential for synthesis of bile acids and nucleic acid.
- The simplest and sweetest of amino acids and is used as a sweetener.

Therapeutic uses
- No proven individual therapeutic uses but together with other amino acids may be useful in conditions of muscular degeneration, skin and connective tissue regeneration and epilepsy.

Proline

- An important component of muscle and collagen (connective tissue).
- Vitamin C is essential for its incorporation into these supporting structures of the body.
- Essential for skin health.

Ornithine

- Important metabolically but not incorporated into protein.
- A very powerful stimulator of growth hormone production by the pituitary gland.

- Increases body metabolism of fat and enhances transportation of amino acids to cells.
- Involved with arginine in ammonia detoxification in the urea cycle.

Therapeutic uses
- Enhances wound healing and stimulates the immune system.
- May be useful in auto-immune diseases such as rheumatoid arthritis.

Threonine

- This essential amino acid is deficient in grains.
- Found abundantly in pulses, making a combination of grain and pulses a complete source of protein for vegetarians.
- Required for digestive and intestinal tract function.
- Prevents accumulation of fat in the liver.
- Suggested to be essential for mental health.

Therapeutic uses
- No specific therapeutic roles have been ascribed to it thus far.

Deficiency
- Irritability and personality disorders.
- Indigestion, malabsorption, malnourishment.

Genetically acquired disorders
- Hyperthreonineaemia, for which there is no adequate treatment.

4 AMINO ACIDS IN ACTION: THE POWER AND THE POTENTIAL

In this section, we shall look at those conditions where amino acids can normalize biochemical imbalances and thus facilitate healing. The replenishment of a deficiency, or rebalancing of an imbalanced ratio between nutrients, simply allows the normal functions of the body, which include its capacity for repair and healing, to operate more efficiently. In certain instances, though, specific pharmacological effects are achieved over and above the replacing of deficient nutrients. DLPA (D and L phenylalanine) or tryptophan is used this way, in pain control treatment. Where possible the text will note this difference in therapeutic use.

While the emphasis of this book is on the role of amino acids in healing, it should go without saying that many other factors are involved in ill health apart from amino acids. Amino acids should never be seen as the only way in which the body should receive assistance. Underlying causes should always be sought and removed or dealt with as appropriate. Nutrition is not the only factor causing disease and dysfunction, although it is one of the most potent influences, and has a part to play in almost every condition, since it can improve the underlying health of the individual and hence help speed recovery.

We need to pay attention to the individuals with the complaint, and all the variables which make them unique, including their nutritional needs, rather than just to the condition. Anyone who treats all headaches, or all stomach aches, or all asthma attacks, for example, with a standard approach is practising bad medicine, as these can all have different causes.

Why then have we, in this section, chosen to present the evidence for the power and potential of amino acids in a format which emphasizes the usefulness related to specific conditions; which does just what we suggest should not be done, and looks at particular health complaints, and what individual amino acids (and other nutrients) can do for them? The reason is simple.

The only other way of presenting evidence would be by describing a long series of individual case histories, showing how amino acids and other nutrients were selected in particular cases, to meet specific and unique needs, rather than dealing just with the symptoms (insomnia, hypertension etc). This would be a preferable way of assessing amino acids. However, were case histories of that sort to be used to illustrate the usefulness of amino acids in therapy, they would be labelled by detractors as being merely anecdotal evidence which 'proves nothing'. This is because of the current medical vogue which pays attention only to trials dealing with diseases or conditions rather than the requirements of individual patients. The various types of 'acceptable' study are explained below.

A group of people with a particular condition are all treated in the same way, and are then compared with another group of people with the same condition, who received dummy (placebo) medication. This is called a **placebo controlled trial**. The people receiving the dummy treatment (or no treatment at all in some instances) are called the **control** group. If the medical staff administering such a trial are unaware of which patients are receiving the real medicine, and which the dummy, the trial would be called a **double blind, placebo controlled trial**; double blind as neither the patient nor the doctor knows whether or not the patient is taking a medicine, nutrient or a dummy, until after the study is completed and benefits (if any) are analysed.

In some studies, the people taking the medicine (or nutrient) are switched half way through the trial, so that they then receive the placebo (and those on the placebo start to receive the 'real' medicine). This is then called a **double blind, placebo controlled, cross-over trial**. In yet another variation the patient is assigned to the placebo or the 'real medicine' group haphazardly, in a random manner, and this is then called a **'randomized' trial**. We might then end up with a **double blind, randomized,**

cross-over, placebo controlled trial. At the end of such studies the results are analysed and the researchers decide whether or not they are statistically 'significant'.

These terms will be used in the text and should be understood to indicate the type of trial performed and whether or not the benefits were statistically better than those which might result from mere chance. It should be noted that in some instances, placebos do better, statistically, than the drug being tested, even in some very serious conditions. The research studies discussed in the text will give the reader an understanding of the ways in which the evidence was gathered. Anyone who wishes to have a deeper understanding of the biochemistry of amino acids and the amazing complexity of their interactions with each other and with the other nutrients and enzymes which allow the body to function, should refer to the books listed in the Resources section. The main objective in writing this book is to promote an understanding of the potential of amino acids as powerful aids to healing.

ALCOHOL DAMAGE AND CRAVING

One of the most serious side effects of excessive alcohol consumption is the damage to the liver. Recent studies have indicated that as little as a glass and a half of wine, or a pint of beer, is regarded as the maximum safe daily intake beyond which damage begins to occur.

Carnitine was studied in an animal trial in which rats were fed an enormous 36 per cent of their total calory intake as ethanol. They developed, not surprisingly, massive liver damage (hepatic steatosis) involving accumulation of fatty acids, cholesterol, phospholipids, triglycerides etc.

When they were given supplements of carnitine, as well as its precursors lysine and methionine, it was found that the carnitine supplemented rats developed significantly less fatty degeneration of the liver than those not supplemented. No advantage was noted in adding the lysine and methionine. The findings suggest that chronic alcoholics have a functional deficiency of carnitine.[1]

NOTE: Animal studies are considered by the author to be undesirable for many reasons, not least of which is the suffering inflicted on the unwilling participants. There is also the very real fact that species are different in the ways in which they react to substances and foods. The animal studies presented in this book should be viewed as merely supporting evidence and not as conclusive findings, which human studies might represent.

In another trial, the use of *mixed free form amino acids* was studied in the treatment of 35 patients with alcoholic hepatitis. Half (17) received a high protein (100 g daily), high calory (3000kcal) diet and between 70 and 85 g of free form amino acids in a balanced mixture. The symptoms of those treated in this way were much improved after a month, with none of these seriously ill individuals dying. The other 18 patients with similar conditions received the same diet but no amino acids, and whilst there was some improvement in this group due to better dietary patterns than previously, it was not as great as in the group treated with amino acids, and four of these 'control' patients died in the month of the study.[2]

A study at Johns Hopkins University School of Medicine showed that patients with acute alcoholic hepatitis (liver disease) had depressed levels of most of the essential and non-essential

amino acids at the time of hospitalization. A similar, but less pronounced, pattern of amino acid deficiency was noted in alcoholics
without liver disease, very similar to those found in African or
Asian famine victims, due to dietary protein deficiency.

When alcohol was stopped, a diet which included protein at a
level of between 1 and 2 g of protein per kilogram of body weight
daily was introduced. This pattern improved the amino acid
status of the alcoholics with liver disease but failed to normalize
such levels as compared with non-alcoholics, despite cessation of
alcohol consumption and an adequate diet. It was found that
despite simultaneous supplementation of vitamin B6 (pyridoxine) the levels of its derivative known as PLP
(pyridoxal-5'-phosphate) failed to normalize in these individuals.
It is known that unless PLP levels approach normal, amino acid
metabolism is altered and absorption and transportation of
amino acids from the bowel are reduced.

*This makes a strong case for supplementation with free form amino acids
as opposed to a simple increase in protein intake, in individuals with severely
compromised biochemistry due to alcohol abuse.*

Supplementation of PLP intravenously until normal function
is achieved may also be called for in such cases.[3]

Glutamine was found to *dramatically diminish the craving for alcohol*
in nine out of 10 patients supplemented with 2 g daily of
glutamine in divided doses.

The patients, their friends and families all stated that there was
a reduction in the craving for alcohol as well as less anxiety and
better sleep.

This was a cross-over study, and it was found that three of the
patients continued to respond to the placebo after glutamine was
stopped, but no patient who started on the placebo produced
positive results.[4]

The distinguished researcher Professor Roger Williams states
that this ability of glutamine to check a craving (e.g. for sugar or
alcohol) probably relates to its effect on the appetite centre in the
brain. He suggests an intake of 2 to 4 g daily.[5]

Drs Janice Phelps and Alan Nourse in their book *The Hidden
Addiction*[6] present a programme for treatment of *alcohol addiction*
and note that as part of the programme *free form amino acid complex
(all the amino acids) should be given in doses of 500 to 1000 mg three times
daily with vitamin B6 (100 mg) to be taken an hour before meals on an*

empty stomach. They too recommend glutamine in a dose of 500 to 1000mg four times daily between meals.

Additional nutrients in their programme include vitamin C, 8 g daily; vitamin B3 (niacinamide) 3 g; pantothenic acid (vitamin B5), 1500 mg daily; vitamin B6 with the amino acids and additionally as a diuretic (caution: doses of B6 in the quantities which they recommend, in excess of a gram a day, could produce neurological symptoms of peripheral neuritis). They also prescribe adrenal cortex extract. In addition they suggest phenylalanine, tyrosine and tryptophan for symptoms of depression and insomnia which might accompany withdrawal from alcohol. These will be discussed when depression and insomnia are considered later in this section.

Dr Robert Erdmann and Meirion Jones in their book *The Amino Revolution*[7] outline a programme for *alcohol addiction* involving *complete free form amino acid, glutamine, glycine, tryptophan and phenylalanine. In addition co-factors such as vitamins B3, B12, C, zinc, selenium and what are termed catabolic amino acids, methionine, taurine and aspartic acid are recommended.*

This latter suggestion (catabolic amino acids) relates to different phases of the metabolic process in which energy release occurs in response to the breakdown of protein structures. Thus the time of day at which nutrients are taken, which affect these and other processes (which are tied to our 'body clocks'), is important. Catabolic nutrients should be taken between 4 and 10pm. For dosage recommendations and discussion of this concept (based on the work of a noted New York physician, Emanuel Revici MD) refer to the Erdmann/Jones book.

References
[1] Sachan, D. et al. *Carnitine and alcohol induced fatty degeneration of the liver*, American Journal of Clinical Nutrition, 39:738–44, 1984.
[2] Nasrallah, S. *Amino acid therapy in alcoholic hepatitis*, The Lancet, 2:1276–7, 1980.
[3] Diehl, A. et al. *Plasma amino acids in alcoholics*, American Journal of Clinical Nutrition, 44:453–60, 1986.
[4] Rogers, L. et al. Quarterly Journal of Studies on Alcohol, 18(4):581–7, 1957.
[5] Williams, R. *Nutrition against Disease*, Bantam Books, 1981.
[6] Phelps, J. and Nourse, A. *The Hidden Addiction*, Little Brown, 1986.
[7] Erdmann, R. and Jones, M. *The Amino Revolution*, Century, 1987.

ABOUT ASPARTAME (NUTRASWEET)

Amino acids are used in many commercial processes, a recent example being as artificial sweeteners for food.

Dr Michael Weiner, author of *Maximum Immunity,* discusses the harmful effects on the immune function of the amino acid combination marketed as the sweetener NutraSweet or aspartame.[1] Once ingested in a cold drink or artificially sweetened food, aspartame, Weiner informs us, breaks down into its constituents, the amino acids phenylalanine and aspartic acid, and the following sequence occurs. 'Methanol (wood alcohol) is formed. Many foods in nature contain methanol, including drinking alcohol, but most sources of methanol in nature are accompanied by ethanol, and it turns out that ethanol is a specific antidote for methanol.' Weiner points out that, when metabolized in the body, methanol (which remember is the end product of aspartame or NutraSweet) becomes the highly poisonous and immune suppressing substance formaldehyde (used for embalming bodies).

If methanol was accidentally consumed, the standard procedure would be to pump the stomach and then to get the individual to consume a large amount of ethanol, making him or her more than slightly drunk. By saturating the system with ethanol in this way, methanol is degraded into acetaldehyde, resulting in drunkenness and a hangover—preferable to death which could result were the methanol allowed simply to degrade into formaldehyde. When Nutrasweet is consumed in sweets, soft drinks etc there is unlikely to be any counterbalancing ethanol intake to allow the relatively safe degradation into acetaldehyde.

Thus, as Weiner points out, the only safe way to consume anything containing this undesirable sweetener would be to accompany it with an alcoholic beverage, not perhaps the best prospect for the health and immune system of a three-year-old who happened to be eating an ice-cream sweetened with aspartame!

Further dangers of the use of aspartame are highlighted by the internationally renowned researcher Professor Richard Wurtman of the Massachusetts Institute of Technology. In a report he shows that a number of neurochemical changes may result from its use, with serious potential consequences. In rats aspartame was shown to double the levels of phenylalanine in the brain, which effect was redoubled when carbohydrates (sugars) were consumed at the same time. This combination raised the levels of tyrosine (which derives from phenylalanine) in the brain by over 300 per cent! There was coincidental depression (by 50 per cent) of the normal increase in brain levels of tryptophan, which would usually follow ingestion of carbohydrates. The amount of sweetener used in this study was equivalent to that consumed by a normal North American child on a hot afternoon (soft drinks, sweets, ices etc). The full implications of such effects on the brains of children were not clear at the time of the study, but subsequent correspondence from Professor Wurtman on the subject indicates that the anxiety felt by many was justified.[2]

Writing to *The Lancet*, Professor Wurtman describes the possibility of a link between seizures (fits) in healthy adults and the use of aspartame. He describes three cases in which the association is assumed. In one a 42-year-old woman drank $3\frac{3}{4}$ litres of diet soda daily. She experienced mood swings, depression and headaches, along with nausea. Ultimately she had seizures (epilepsy).

A second case involved a 27-year-old male who drank four or five glasses of diet (non-sugar and sweetened with aspartame) drink daily. He developed twitches at night along with abnormal breathing, a severe headache and eventually grand mal seizures (epileptic fits). The third case involved a 36-year-old man who drank nearly a litre daily of aspartame-sweetened tea. He too developed seizures. *In all cases headaches and other symptoms disappeared after aspartame sweetened drinks were stopped.*

In his letter, Wurtman described a sequence of events as involving increased levels of phenylalanine, leading to abnormal levels of catocholamine and serotonin production in the brain, due to imbalances caused by the absence of other neutral amino acids. This would set the scene for the sort of symptoms listed above.[3]

It is as well to consider that in certain instances the use of supplemental amino acids could cause imbalances similar to this, unless strict attention is paid to the guidelines given as to dosage etc. Because something is helpful it does not mean that more of the same will be better. This is especially true of some of the amino acids which sometimes work therapeutically in small amounts, and not in large ones. If advice given in this book is followed, then there will be no such dangers. Please follow the guidelines and doses recommended.

References

[1] Weiner, M. *Maximum Immunity,* Gateway Books, Bath, 1987.
[2] Wurtman, R. New England Journal of Medicine, 309:249, 1983.
[3] Wurtman, R. Letter to The Lancet, 8463:1060, 1985.

ATHEROSCLEROSIS AND CARDIOVASCULAR/ CIRCULATORY PROBLEMS

There is no suggestion intended that amino acids alone are the answer to these conditions. However, they form a major element in the pathology of damaged cardiovascular structures, and can be important in their healing. Cardiovascular and circulatory problems kill more people than any other disease in industrialized societies, and have many dietary causes including *excessive intake* of hydrogenated (saturated) fats, mainly of animal origin, excess intake of refined carbohydrate, excess cholesterol levels in the system, *low levels* of selenium, vitamin C, specific essential fatty acids (such as omega 3 and omega 6), potassium, chromium, vitamin E etc.

A diet low in animal fat, cholesterol, alcohol, caffeine and refined carbohydrate, high in complex carbohydrates (vegetables, fruits, beans, wholegrains etc) and supplemented as indicated with nutrients, especially vitamins B, C and E, the essential fatty acids, and calcium, magnesium, chromium, selenium, zinc, coenzyme Q_{10} etc, will help to enhance cardio-vascular function if used alongside the amino acids discussed below. Herbal products such as ginger and garlic are also noted as being useful in supplying essential nutrients and having beneficial actions on the circulatory function. Smoking should also be avoided.[1][2][3]

A human study showed that individuals consuming a diet high in animal protein, whose blood levels of the amino acids *lysine* were in a ratio of 3.5 to 1 or higher in relation to *arginine* were at much *higher risk of arteriosclerosis* due to excessive levels of *lysine*. Vegetarians have been shown to have a much lower ratio of these two amino acids than meat eaters, and consequently a lower incidence of arteriosclerosis. The ratio of lysine to arginine in meat is between 3 and 4 to 1, whereas in plant proteins it is between 1 and 1.25 to 1.[4]

In a double blind, cross-over study 44 men with *stable, chronic angina* which appeared after exercise were given either *L-carnitine* (1 g twice daily) or a placebo. After a month, it was found that the patients receiving carnitine could take more exercise without inducing pain, whereas the placebo group remained unaltered.[5]

Italian research has shown that during *acute or chronic cardiac ischemia* (lack of oxygen reaching the heart muscle, often due to arteriosclerosis) there was both a deficiency of *carnitine* in these tissues and an accumulation of various fatty substances which carnitine is able to deactivate. Patients who had died of *acute myocardial infarction* were shown to have gross deficiency of *carnitine* in the heart muscles. It was suggested by the researchers that were adequate carnitine available in the body, the tissues could have been restored to normal.[6]

One Japanese study involved 62 patients suffering from *congestive heart failure*. This was a double blind, randomized, crossover, placebo controlled trial, in which the amino acid *taurine* was supplied in three daily doses of 2 g each for four weeks. After four weeks the patients receiving taurine showed many *significant improvements* including better breathing, fewer palpitations, less swelling (oedema), improved laboratory and X-ray evidence as to heart status, and an overall improvement in function (by the New York Heart Association functional classification) which simply meant that the patients receiving taurine could do more than previously and than the placebo group.

It was also found that patients receiving taurine could reduce their medication intake (digitalis and/or diuretics).

Neither heart rate nor blood pressure was affected by taurine intake. Taurine is known to be the most abundant free amino acid found in healthy cardiac tissues. The researchers concluded that taurine may be a useful agent that could be given by itself, or along with more conventional forms of therapy, for the treatment of congestive heart failure.[7].

In a study of 97 consecutive patients with *acute chest pains* it was found that those patients suffering *myocardial infarction (heart attacks)* had much higher levels of *taurine* being selectively 'leaked' into the bloodstream from the heart muscles. The requirement for taurine at such a time is very great and the normal supply became depleted, leading to its withdrawal.

The researchers noted that it acts in the same way as magnesium, having a *direct effect on the levels of potassium which pass into and out of the heart muscle cells*, a most important element in its health.[8][9]

The importance of *taurine* in *maintaining normal electrical and mechanical activity of the heart muscle* is shown in animal studies involving rats and guinea pigs. The electrolytic state of the heart was normalized by use of taurine when artificial damage was created in these animals by a variety of means.[10] [11]

A study of the effectiveness of *tryptophan* in the treatment of *cardiac conditions* revealed that its ability to produce a relaxation of muscle tone *lowered the incidence of anticipated deaths from heart attacks by 15 per cent*. This effect was achieved by reducing the likelihood of heart spasm, racing heart rate and fibrillation (uncontrolled fluttering of the heart muscles).[12]

An animal study (using rabbits and rats) was conducted using *glycine, arginine and alanine* to see the effects on *reduction of increased levels of cholesterol*. These were artificially induced through dietary manipulation. It was found that arginine and alanine supplementation reduced serum cholesterol of rabbits by 20 per cent. When glycine was added, levels of cholesterol were halved.

The size and number of atherosclerotic lesions in the animals' aortas were reduced as the cholesterol levels came down with amino acid supplementation. The serum levels of cholesterol of rats were reduced by half when glycine was added. When casein (milk solids) was replaced with soy protein, cholesterol levels were reduced by two thirds. Excessive intake of casein also results in an imbalance in amino acid levels, which is beneficially affected by glycine and possibly arginine and alanine. The human implications of this study are not immediately clear except that a great many people ingest heroic amounts of dairy produce, which is known to have negative effects on atherosclerosis.[13]

In addition to the specific effects of amino acids reported above, methionine may be useful (in combination with an appropriate cholesterol reducing diet) in preventing arteriosclerosis (hardening of the arteries). This sulphur rich amino acid, vital for the production of certain enzymes which *protect the arterial wall*, also acts as a *detoxifier of heavy metals* (via a physiological method called chelation in which it literally grabs the metal atoms and removes them from the scene). It is also a *powerful antioxidant*.

A number of other nutrient co-factors are required to act with methionine for it to work efficiently, including vitamin B6 (pyridoxine). We should also recall (see Chapter 3) that methionine (or lysine) becomes carnitine in the presence of adequate vitamin C.

Colin Goodliffe recommends a dosage of 600 to 2000 mg daily of car-

nitine to raise levels of beneficial lipoproteins and to lower cholesterol levels.[14] *Robert Erdmann and Meirion Jones maintain that a cocktail of nutrients should be employed to achieve maximum heart health, both in a protective and therapeutic setting. These include individual amounts of methionine, serine, tryptophan and histidine as well as a complete blend of free form amino acids. Co-factors such as vitamins B3 (niacin), B5 (pantothenic acid), B6 (pyridoxine), B12 (cynaocobalamine) and folic acid, vitamins C and E, magnesium and zinc are also recommended. For the rationale of this approach read* The Amino Revolution *by Robert Erdmann PhD and Meirion Jones (see Recommended Reading, page 122).*

References

[1] Davies, S. and Stewart, A. *Nutritional Medicine*, Pan Books, 1987.

[2] Warbach, M. *Nutritional Influences on Illness*, Third Line Press, California, 1987.

[3] Goodliffe, C. *How to Avoid Heart Disease*, Blandford Press, Poole, 1987.

[4] Sanchez, A. *Nutrition Reports International*, 28:497, 1983.

[5] Cherchi, A. et al. *Carnitine effect on exercise tolerance in chronic stable angina*, International Journal of Clinical Pharmacology and Therapeutic Toxicology, 23(10):569-72, 1985.

[6] The Lancet, Vol 1:1419-20, 1982.

[7] Azuma, J. et al. *Taurine and congestive heart failure*, Circulation Research, 34(4):543-57, 1983.

[8] Lombardini, J. et al. *Elevated blood taurine levels in acute myocardial infarction*, Journal of Laboratory and Clinical Medicine, 98(6):849-59, 1981.

[9] Chazov, E.' et al. *Taurine and electrical activity of heart*, Circulation Research, 35 (suppl) 3:11-21, 1974.

[10] Shustova, T. et al. *Effect of Taurine on potassium, calcium, and sodium levels in the blood and tissues of rats*, Jn Vopr. Med. Khim., 32(4):113-16, 1986.

[11] Franconi, F. et al. *Protective effect of taurine on hypoxia*, Biochemical Pharmacology, 34(15):2611-15, 1985.

[12] Sved, A. et al. *Studies of anti-hypertensive action of L tryptophan*, Journal of Pharmacological and Experimental Therapeutics, 221: 329-33, 1982.

[13] Katan, M. et al. *Reduction in casein-induced hypercholesterolaemia and atherosclerosis in rabbits and rats by dietary glycine, arginine and alanine*, Atherosclerosist, 43:381, 1982.

[14] Goodliffe, C. *How to Avoid Heart Disease*, Blandford Press, Poole, 1987.

BEHAVIOUR MODIFICATION FOR AGGRESSION

As neurotransmitters are heavily involved in brain and nervous system function, and as amino acids are essential to neurotransmitters (see page 25), then it follows that behaviour might be modified when these are imbalanced, either in excess or deficient. There is abundant evidence linking aggressive, anti-social behaviour with nutrient imbalances and with heavy metal toxicity (lead, mercury, cadmium, aluminium etc).

Alexander Schauss has shown that nutritional modification can alter aggressive juvenile delinquent behaviour dramatically. Among his findings were that many aggressive individuals were sensitive to specific foods, most notably dairy produce, and that removal of the offending food improved behaviour. In terms of toxicity he notes that the amino acids methionine, cysteine and cystine all contain sulphur compounds which naturally latch onto (chelate) toxic metals in the body and help in their removal (vitamin C, calcium, zinc and pectin also help in this process).[1]

Dr Stephen Levine, director of research for the Allergy Research Group, states that there is now considerable interest in how imbalances between two or more neuroregulators may cause behavioural disorders. There has been some research into the relationship between inadequate serotonin (derived from tryptophan in the body) and aggressive behaviour. Studies have reported that reduced levels of serotonin in the brain result in aggressive behaviour, and that low levels of norepinephrine and high levels of dopamine (both of which derive from phenylalanine and tyrosine) increase aggressive behaviour.[2]

It has also been shown that when there is a lot of tryptophan in the diet, and the balance is high, compared with other amino acids, feelings of fatigue and inertia are reported.[3]

Recent experiments on rats have shown the link between aggression and tryptophan. When tryptophan was deliberately eliminated from the diet of these animals they became extremely aggressive and murdered each other (this is known as muricide in scientific jargon). This behaviour was stopped when tryptophan was added to the diet.[4]

As a result of this type of research tryptophan has been used on aggressive schizophrenic patients. Female schizophrenics have been shown to be low in tryptophan and their levels have increased with recovery.[5]

In an experimental double blind cross-over study, 12 male patients alternately received either a placebo or a dosage of tryptophan. The patients with a large number of aggressive incidents improved on tryptophan. Their hostility also lessened and their mood improved. Those patients who had no such aggressive history worsened on tryptophan supplementation.[6]

References
[1] Schauss, A. *Diet, Crime and Delinquency*, Parker House, California, 1980.
[2] Levine, S. *Behavioural Ecology*, Bioscience, Vol. 2 Nos. 5&6.
[3] Wurtman, R. The Lancet, May 21 1983 p1145.
[4] Broderick, P. Lynch, V. *Behavioural and biochemical changes induced by lithium and tryptophan*, Neuropharmacology, 21:6671, 1982.
[5] Gilmour, D. et al. Biological Psychiatry, 6:119, 1973.
[6] Morand, C. et al. Biological Psychiatry, 18:575–8, 1983.

CANDIDA ALBICANS (YEAST OVERGROWTH)

The health problems associated with yeast overgrowth are many and varied and range from genito-urinary disorders to digestive bloating and emotional instability, including depression, anxiety and phobic behaviour (see my book, *Candida Albicans, Could Yeast be Your Problem?* Thorsons, 1986).

The increase in Candida activity in recent years has been ascribed to a number of factors: increased use of antibiotics (which kill friendly bacteria in the gut, a normal part of the controlling mechanism against yeast spread); use of hormone drugs such as the contraceptive pill, which enhances yeast activity; and a dietary pattern rich in sugars, which yeast thrives on.

A variety of nutritional controlling strategies have been devised, including a low sugar diet coupled with the use of high-potency acidophilus cultures (superdophilus etc) to repopulate the bowel with friendly bacteria, the taking of garlic, olive oil (for oleic acid), the B vitamin biotin as well as aloe vera juice, and the trace element germanium, all of which have anti-candida potential. Specific anti-candida drugs, such as nystatin and caprystatin (a derivative of coconut), are often used.

Because of malabsorption and maldigestion problems, which are often associated with Candida activity, the use of a full range of free form amino acids is often suggested to enhance overall nutritional balance.

One of the problems in diagnosing Candida activity has been the fact that every man, woman and child in the world is host to this yeast, and it is therefore sometimes hard to know whether or not it is out of control and causing the types of symptoms described above. When Candida is out of control and rampant, amino acid profiles have, however, been shown to have distinctive patterns. When Candida is active, the following substances are usually found to be present in relatively large amounts in the urine: *phosphoserine, beta-alanine, gamma-aminobutyric acid, hydroxylysine, ornithine, anserine, carnosine,* phosphoethanolamine, ethanolamine, 1-methylhistidine, 3-methylhistidine, ammonia. The first seven of these (in italics) are not usually even detectable in urine (anserine is not even found in human tissues) and their presence indicates that they are the result of unusual activity in the body, or that they are by-products of yeast activity.

These findings were compared with profiles of other patients, not affected by Candida, and were found to be distinctive. Very low levels of arginine were measured in 96 per cent of Candida patients. The researcher in this study states that, 'These high levels of amino acids occur simultaneously and suggest metabolic disorders involving phospholipid metabolism, liver, kidney, maldigestion, malabsoption, connective tissue, and pyridoxal-5'-phosphate (vitamin B6) metabolism.'[1]

What is fascinating is that when Candida is treated successfully by the methods outlined above, the changing pattern can be read on subsequent amino acid profiles, giving the doctor an objective method of assessing progress. Amino acid profiles are available in the UK and USA, see Resources, page 121).

References

[1] Traister, J. *Abnormal aminoaciduria pattern diagnosed with candidiasis,* Paper presented at meeting of American Society of Clinical Pathologists, Orlando, Florida Sept 27 1986.

CATARACTS

Over half the population over the age of 65 in the USA are affected by cataracts, and these are a major cause of blindness in Africa. They occur when ultra-violet light produces the development of free radicals which damage the lens.

A number of connections have been made between the development of cataracts and diet. Among the main causes are excessive sugar intake and high levels of dairy produce (mainly milk), as well as deficiencies (and excess) of the B vitamin riboflavin (B2). It has been suggested that people with cataracts should have no more than 10 mg daily of riboflavin in supplement form. Zinc may also be deficient.

The antioxidant nutrients vitamin C (which should be present at 30 to 50 times its normal level in the bloodstream), vitamin E, and the mineral selenium are found to be helpful in retarding the damage to the eye caused by what are called 'free radicals'. These are minute destructive biochemical entities which occur when molecules with unpaired electrons cause a chain reaction of cell damage, leading, depending upon the location, to changes such as the onset of arterial disease or even cancer, and in this case to cataracts. Antioxidants prevent this damage.[1]

Amino acids contain a number of important antioxidants, and those which are particularly effective in cataract treatment are cysteine and methionine levels of which decrease with age. Plentiful supply of both of these is essential for the synthesis of glutathione peroxidase, the main defender of the eye against the sort of damage induced by free radicals. Selenium is also important in this process.

An article in the *Journal of the American Medical Association* discusses the relationship between cataracts and a lack of glutathione peroxidase, and suggests that decline in glutathione peroxidase can be halted by diets rich in cysteine and methionine.[2]

Dr Alex Duarte has traced the mechanism of lens physiology, and has researched into the nutrients involved in cataract development. He points out that the enzymes hexokinase and phosphofructokinase are responsible for the energy production which keeps the so-called 'lens cation pump' mechanism active. This pumps sodium out and potassium in to the lens, thus maintaining high levels of amino acids for the synthesis of protein. If the energy supply becomes diminished, this pump mechanism slowly fails, resulting in loss of protein synthesis, loss of transparency, and hardening of the lens proteins, which change from being 80 per cent soluble to being only 35 per cent soluble in a lens with a cataract. Duarte also points to glutathione peroxidase as a major form of protection against this process, and suggests that treatment consisting of a combination of amino acids, enzymes and vitamins could correct the various imbalances.

This approach is claimed to be 80 per cent effective in slowing or stopping progression of senile cataracts. Trials in Bonn have demonstrated the safety and efficacy of this method through both double blind trials and animal studies. Of interest is the fact that it is normal for the concentration of vitamin C in the lens to be 30 to 50 times the level found in the bloodstream. This is vital for protecting the lens.

The aim in treatment is not to restore damaged tissues but to normalize energy production in the eye and thus stabilize the operating mechanisms, improve protein synthesis and eventually retard the degenerative process. The nutrients used are combined in a French product now available in the USA and called 'C-Thru'. It is marketed by D&B Enterprises, 19400 Beach Boulevard, Suite 21, Huntington Beach, California 92647.[3]

Cysteine and methionine are sulphur rich amino acids and are found in eggs, beans, garlic and onions. However since it takes a great deal of any of these foods to make a significant contribution to the body's levels of amino acids it is suggested that supplements should also be taken.

Dosage for methionine is between 200 and 1000 mg daily, with water, away from mealtimes (no closer than 90 minutes to any protein intake or absorption of the amino acid will be impaired).

Dosage for cysteine is between 1 and 2 g daily with vitamin C at the same time at a level of three times the amount of C to cysteine. Cysteine should also be taken away from mealtimes with water.

NOTE: Cysteine should not be given to diabetics without professional guidance.

References
[1] Werbach, M. *Nutritional Influences On Illness,* Third Line Press, California, 1987.

[2] Cole, H. *Enzyme activity may hold key to cataract activity,* Journal of the American Medical Association 254(8):1008, 1985.

[3] Duarte, A. *Cataracts can be stopped without surgery,* Health Consciousness 5(4), 1984.

CHRONIC DISEASE (MENTAL OR PHYSICAL)

William Philpott MD has conducted extensive research into the deficiencies that cause chronic ill health. He makes the following claim: 'Our statistical study reveals that the majority of degenerative illnesses, whether physical or mental, have a vitamin B6 utilization disorder...it seems evident that one of the problems producing B6 utilization disorder is low cystine (cysteine)...Cystine is a necessary amino acid which the body makes from the essential amino acid methionine...the universality of cystine not being formed from methionine in chronic degenerative diseases suggests that a state of addiction or toxins associated with addiction, interferes with methionine metabolism.'

Philpott's answer to this is to supplement all cases of chronic degenerative disease with cystine or cysteine at doses of 1½ g, three times daily for a month, with dosage then reduced to twice daily. In addition he suggests 50 mg of pyridoxal-5'-phosphate (the active form of vitamin B6) three times daily. Philpott further points out that the most commonly deficient substance noted in amino acid profiles of people with degenerative diseases is the precursor of glumatic acid, alpha-ketoglutaric acid. This is associated with vitamin B6 in many enzyme activities. Glumatic acid is also shown to be invariably low in these very sick people.

Philpott notes that the major body cycles of detoxification and energy production are linked by the amino acid, aspartic acid. In a complex set of biochemical steps he finds that supplementation of aspartic acid and citric acid helps to normalize the cycles and restore balance to many of these imbalances.

Dosages of 500 mg aspartic acid and 750 mg citric acid are suggested five times daily (on rising, at each meal and on retiring). If resulting digestive discomfort is noted, he recommends a quarter teaspoon of bicarbonate of soda as well.[1]

References
[1] Information sheets, Philpott Medical Center, Oklahoma City, 1983.

DEPRESSION

There are many causes of depression. Many cases have been shown to relate to alterations in the body's biochemistry, although not in any uniform pattern. The disorder appears either as depression alone (uni-polar) or (far more seriously) in the form of mood swings from manic behaviour to deep depression (bi-polar). Manic behaviour involves violent, often aggressive, physical activity, restlessness, and the feeling of being mentally supercharged. Depression is characterized by exhaustion and a withdrawal from any form of activity and involvement.

These conditions are known as affective disorders, and the biochemical alterations which take place may relate to specific deficiencies or to excess amounts of toxic substances including heavy metals (eg vanadium) and sometimes of normally safe nutrients. For example, cases are reported of mania (insomnia, delusions and excessive energy etc) developing when large quantities of glutamine (2 to 4 g daily) were ingested.[1]

In one study of 40 patients with *major depression* of whom eight were bi-polar depressives, *L-phenylalanine (LPA)* (the precursor of tyrosine) was given. Dosage was *500 mg in the morning and again at noon, plus vitamin B6* (100 mg twice daily), for a week at the outset. Phenylalanine was then *increased by 500 mg daily until benefits (or side effects) were noted*, with a maximum intake of 4 g daily.

Thirty-one of the patients *improved almost immediately*, including seven of the eight bi-polar depressives. It was suggested that most of the others who found benefit were marginally tending towards bi-polar symptoms and that phenylalanine was more beneficial in such cases. Ten of the patients were completely free of depressive symptoms after supplementation.

Side effects of slight headache of short duration, constipation, slight nausea and insomnia were noted in some patients.[2 3]

In treatment *D-phenylalanine* was also effective in relieving depressive symptoms in cases of plain depression without manic tendencies.[4]

In a double blind controlled study 14 *depressed* patients were given *DL-phenylalanine (DLPA)* in doses of *150 to 200 mg daily* while another group of patients (controls) received an anti-depressive drug (imipramine). At the end of the month's study no difference could be noted between the two groups, showing that *DLPA was at least as effective as the drug.*[5]

Arnold Fox MD, in his book *DLPA: The Natural Pain Killer and Anti-Depressant* (see Recommended Reading, page 121), takes a strongly nutritional approach to the care of depression, including supplementing DL-phenylalanine and tryptophan.

He sees the effects of DLPA on depression to be the result of three factors:

1. Increased levels of norepinephrine which relieves depression (the 'D' form appears the most likely cause here as it is less likely to be harnessed by the body for other uses than is the 'L' form).

2. Increased levels of phenylethylamine (PEA) which is a neurotransmitter closely linked to norepinephrine. Depressed individuals have very low levels of PEA, which antidepressive drugs tend to raise.

3. Increased manufacture of endorphins (literally *endo*genous (self-produced) *morphines*) which act to produce feelings of euphoria.

Apart from a range of vitamins and minerals designed to enhance general function, Fox suggests *500 mg of tryptophan twice daily, at 8am and 8pm, as well as 375 mg of DLPA with breakfast and with lunch. This dosage should be increased to three times daily after a few days. It is to be assumed that these should be taken well before meals rather than with food, although this is not Fox's advice, which goes against the trend of most.*

A variety of studies have been conducted treating both bi-polar and uni-polar disorders with the amino acid tryptophan either alone or in combination with other nutrients.

In an experimental placebo controlled, double blind trial 24 patients with *manic disorders* were treated for seven days with *12 g of tryptophan* daily (this was given in divided doses, without any form of protein 90 minutes before or after it and with a little sugar to enhance its absorption). After a week, half the patients were randomly selected to continue this dosage while the other half were given a placebo. In the second week, *only the patients receiving placebo were seen to display manic symptoms.*[6]

Tryptophan is more effective if also taken with vitamin B6 (pyridoxine).[7] In uni-polar depression *doses of 4 to 6 g of tryptophan daily* (divided doses away from protein and with sugar) are seen to be more helpful than higher or lower doses.[8]

Studies show that *depressive patients* have *low levels of tryptophan* in their bloodstreams as compared with normal individuals. In one, 50 depressive women with uni-polar depression had lower than average levels of tryptophan. Patients who had recovered from depression also had lower levels than control patients, and those who had recovered without the use of antidepressive drugs had higher, more normal, levels than those who had been treated with drugs. A second study showed that amongst women suffering from post-natal depression, those with the deepest depression were the ones with the lowest levels of tryptophan in their bloodstreams.[9][10]

NOTE: Tryptophan is dangerous if taken at the same time as monoamine oxidase inhibitor drugs (MAO inhibitors) or tricyclics, which are often prescribed to depressed patients because it enhances their side effects. If you are on these, do not take tryptophan without first seeking professional advice.

The amino acid *tyrosine* which derives from phenylalanine has been shown to be *effective in treatment of some cases of uni-polar depression*, taken in doses of 2 g, three times daily. Three out of five such cases, none of whom was receiving other medication, showed a *50 per cent reduction in levels of depression* in a four-week double blind placebo-controlled study. Levels of tyrosine rose in those patients whose depression was observed to improve. The only side effects noted were mild gastric upsets when tyrosine was taken without food.[11]

The trials and studies reported above indicate that *some* patients respond very well to particular amino acid supplementation when depressed or in a state of manic depression. In another study of severely depressed people, 80 per cent experienced relief after taking 100 to 500 mg of L-phenylalanine (which is converted into tyrosine in the liver) daily for a fortnight.[12]

The questions should be addressed, if phenylalanine is as helpful as this, why did the other 20 per cent fail to respond? Is it possible to identify, in advance, which patients will respond beneficially? Much of the answer has been provided by an Australian researcher, Dr Robert Buist. He has observed that some depressed people have low levels of the hormone noradrenaline in the brain (identified by the low levels in their urine of certain biochemical waste products such as MHPG or 3-methoxy-4-hydroxyphenthylene glycol). These people will have responded well to treatment with tricyclic drugs such as imipramine and desipramine, but will have a poor response to amitriptyline. They will also usually respond well to tyrosine supplementation since it is a precursor of noradrenaline. A second group who are biochemically different show normal or high levels of MHPG in their urine indicating high levels of noradrenaline in the brain. They would respond poorly to imipramine (tricyclic drugs) and well to amitriptyline, which tends to raise serotonin levels which are low in such cases. It is therefore possible to know in advance which amino acid will help in particular cases of depression by analysing the urine for MHPG, or by studying previous response to antidepressive drugs. This does of course require expert advice and assessment, and it is unwise to try and diagnose yourself.[13]

It is not surprising that precursors of neurotransmitters, such as the amino acids described in the studies above, should be so helpful. What is amazing is that medical science has taken so long to realize the potential of these amazing nutrients.

A neurotransmitter is a chemical messenger which enhances or retards transmission of nerve impulses as necessary. There are many different neurotransmitters, one of which is serotonin which derives from tryptophan. Others include dopamine and adrenaline which derive from tyrosine and phenylalanine. They are also important in weight control, as will be discussed later in this section.

The levels of serotonin will alter according to the supply of tryptophan or dopamine in the brain, with profound influence on mood and behaviour. High levels of ammonia in the brain affect mood and behaviour and can be removed by supplementation by glutamine.

Other nutrients which can be helpful in cases of depression include most of the B-complex vitamins, vitamin C, calcium, magnesium, zinc, iron, potassium and essential fatty acids (evening primrose oil or vitamin F). Food allergies or sensitivities should also be considered as causes and identified and eliminated.

This may call for periods on a severely restricted diet (the so-called Stone Age diet) and rotation diets which carefully programme consumption of specific food families until culprit foods are identified. Doctors who specialize in this form of treatment are called clinical ecologists.

References

1 Letter to the American Journal of Psychiatry 141, October 10 1984.

2 Sabelli, H. et al. *Clinical studies on the phenylalanine hypothesis of affective disorder*, Journal of Clinical Psychiatry, 47(20):66–70, 1986.

3 *Phenylalanine: A psychoactive nutrient for some depressives?* Medical World News, October 27 1983.

4 Beckmann, H. *Phenylalanine in affective disorders,* Advanced Biological Psychiatry, 10:137–47, 1983.

5 Be⸱ ⸱nn, H. *DLPA versus imipramine,* Arch Psychiatr, Nervenkr, 27: ⸱8, 1979

6 Chouinard, G. et al. *A controlled clinical trial of L-tryptophan in acute mania,* Biological Psychiatry, 20:546–57, 1985.

7 Green, A. et al. *Pharmokinetics of tryptophan* Advanced Biological Psychiatry, 10:67–81, 1983.

8 Wallinder, J. Advanced Biological Psychiatry, 10:82–93, 1983.

9 Coppen, A. *Tryptophan and depressive illness*, Psychological Medicine, 8:49–57, 1978.

10 Stein, G. et al. *Relationship between mood disturbances and tryptophan levels in post-partum women,* British Medical Journal, 2:457, 1976.

11 Gibson, C. *Tyrosine for treatment of depression,* Advanced Biological Psychiatry, 10:148–59, 1983.

12 Gelenberg, A. *Tyrosine for the treatment of depression*, American Journal of Psychiatry, 147:622, 1980.

13 Buist, R. *Therapeutic predictability of tryptophan and tyrosine in treatment of depression,* International Clinical Nutrition Review, 3(2):1–3, 1983.

DIABETES MELLITUS

The amino acids *cysteine, glycine and glutamic acid* (as well as vitamin B3 and the mineral chromium) make up what is known as the glucose tolerance factor (GTF) which is profoundly important in our handling of sugars because they can make the effects of insulin more powerful. This is of great importance to diabetics, and these amino acids as well as the chromium and vitamin B3 may be supplemented, under supervision, thus meaning that intake of additional insulin can be reduced.

Diabetes is a serious condition and any attempt at self-treatment should involve great care. Carbohydrate and fat selection (basically low refined carbohydrate and fat intake and high complex (unrefined) carbohydrate intake) should be low, and *use should be made of a variety of nutrient aids including many of the B vitamins, vitamins C and E, calcium, zinc, magnesium, manganese, phosphorus, potassium, bioflavonoids, coenzyme Q_{10} and the amino acid complex glutathione.*[1]

Glutathione (which is made up of glutamic acid, cysteine and glycine) is suggested for *diabetics* due to its ability to reduce the levels of dehydroascorbic acid, the precursor of vitamin C in red blood cells. Dehydroascorbic acid is increased in diabetics, having, it is thought, harmful effects. Vitamin C is generally in short supply in the plasma of diabetics.[2]

References
[1] Warbach, M. *Nutritional Influences on Illness*, Third Line Press, California, 1987.
[2] Banarjee, S. *Physiological role of dehydroascorbic acid*, Indian Journal of Physiological Pharmacology, 21(2):85–93, 1977.

ENLARGED PROSTATE GLAND (BENIGN PROSTATIC HYPERPLASIA OR BPH)

This condition affects roughly half the male population in industrialized societies, and appears to be largely preventable (and often successfully treatable) using a combination of nutritional approaches, including supplementation with zinc and a selection of amino acids.

The mixture of amino acids reported on in the trials discussed below (glutamic acid, alanine and glycine) were supplemented in two capsules of 1 g each (of the mixture) three times daily for a fortnight, followed by one capsule three times daily.

A study was carried out in which 17 men with *BPH* were supplemented with a mixture of *glumatic acid, alanine and glycine.* It was found that the *retention of urine* (a major problem in BPH) was reduced in eight cases, while the symptom of pain or difficulty in passing urine *(dysuria)* was reduced in 14 cases. All benefits were achieved with no side effects.[1]

In one double blind study, patients were either given the three amino acids as listed above, or glutamic acid and alanine, or glutamic acid alone. Those receiving *all three amino acids* reported *marked subjective improvements in symptoms* as compared with the two control groups. There was however little palpable change in the size of the enlarged prostate noted in any of the patients, with any of the three forms of supplementation.[2]

In a controlled study of 45 patients the *triple amino acid mixture* was supplemented and resulted in 95 per cent of the patients reporting that the symptom of having to pass water during the night *(nocturia) was relieved;* 81 per cent reported *reduced urgency*; 73 per cent reported *reduction in frequency* of urination, while the problem of a long *delay in commencing the flow* when trying to pass water *was relieved* in 70 per cent of cases.[3]

In most cases of BPH, zinc supplementation has been shown to reduce both symptoms and size of the enlarged gland. *Dosage recommended is between 50 and 150 mg daily of zinc gluconate, or if available zinc orotate or zinc picolinate, not taken at mealtimes. In order to avoid the problem of the supplemented zinc interfering with absorption of iron, iron rich foods should be eaten at mealtimes with ½ g to 1 g of vitamin C to enhance its absorption.* Essential fatty acids (also known as vitamin F) such as evening primrose oil or linseed oil have also been found helpful in treating BPH (dosage 1 to 1½ g daily).

WARNING: Other factors (including infection and sometimes malignancy) may enter into enlarged prostate conditions and expert advice should be sought so that an accurate diagnosis is made before self-treatment is attempted.

References

[1] Aito, K. *Conservative treatment of prostatic hypertrophy*, Hinyokika Kiyo, 18(1):41–4, 1972.

[2] Shimaya, M. *Double blind test of PPC for prostatic hyperplasia*, Hinyokika Kiyo, 16(5):231–6, 1970.

[3] Dumrau, F. *BPH: Amino acid therapy for symptomatic relief*, American Journal of Geriatrics,10:426–30, 1962.

EPILEPSY

Epileptic seizures are essentially the result of aberrant neurological discharges in the brain, sometimes apparently due to, or associated with, particular nutrient deficiencies, including vitamin B6 (pyridoxine), magnesium, manganese, zinc, etc.

It is not recommended that people suffering from epilepsy should treat themselves, but rather, that they should seek the advice of a physician who is aware of nutrient connections with the condition. (For how to go about finding one of these, see Resources on page 122.)

Several amino acids have been shown to be effective in the treatment of epilepsy, including taurine and dimethyl glycine.

Studies show low levels of *taurine* (which is a neuroinhibitory agent) *and glutamic acid*, as well as high levels of *glycine*, in those sites in the brain where maximum seizure activity is occurring.[1] *Taurine is therefore recommended in the treatment of epilepsy in doses of 500 mg three times daily, away from protein meals and with water.*[2] Animal studies on rats show that taurine controls experimentally induced seizures. This effect was powerful and of long duration.[3][4]

It appears that taurine works by normalizing the balance of other amino acids, which in epilepsy are thoroughly disordered. Epilepsy causes lowering of serum levels in over half the amino acids, whilst raising those of taurine, except in the cerebrospinal fluid which bathes the brain, where taurine levels are reduced during epileptic seizures. Zinc, which raises serum taurine levels, is low in epileptics.[5]

. *Dimethyl glycine (DMG)*, which is formed in the body when homocysteine is converted into methionine before the formation of glycine, was observed to *reduce seizure frequency* in a male aged 22, who had a long history of generalized epileptic seizures. When supplementation of 90 mg twice daily of DMG was introduced, seizures were reduced from 16 to three a week. On each occasion that DMG was withdrawn the seizures recurred at their previously high level.[6]

NOTE: See also page 50, for the link between epilepsy and the amino acid based artificial sweetener, aspartame.

References
[1] Sherman, J. *Taurine in Nutrition*, Comprehensive Therapy, 35:672, 1979.

[2] Warbach, M. *Nutritional Influences on Illness*, Third Line Press, California, 1987.

[3] Mantovani, J. et al. *Effects of Taurine on Seizures*, Arch Neuro, 35:672, 1979.

[4] Huxtable, R. et al. *Prolonged anticonvulsant action of taurine*, Canadian Journal of Neurological Science, 5:220, 1978.

[5] Chaitow, L. *Amino Acids in Therapy*, Thorsons, 1985.

[6] Roach, E. N. *N-Dimethylglycine for epilepsy,* Letter to the New England Journal of Medicine, 307:1081-2, 1982.

FATIGUE

There are many different causes of fatigue, which is after pain the commonest symptom reported to doctors. There is therefore no obvious simple prescription that can help all types of fatigue, which result from deficiency, toxicity, organic disease (diabetes, cardiac disease etc), chronic pain, obesity, psychosocial problems such as depression, chronic infections, inadequate exercise or sleep, environmental factors such as pollution, lifestyle factors such as smoking, alcohol, drug abuse etc, and many other causes including personality or genetic factors.

There are, however, certain nutritional supplements that can help in most cases of fatigue, including the B-complex vitamins, vitamin C, magnesium, potassium, zinc and a number of the amino acids as listed below. Many of these nutrients assist in the energy manufacturing and detoxification cycles of the body. Two recently researched nutrients, organic germanium and coenzyme Q_{10}, also have a specific relationship to energy. See the Resources section for books about fatigue which give information about the problem; we shall concentrate here on amino acids.

Aspartic acid is a major element in the energy cycle of the body and is therefore a useful supplement to relieve fatigue. Between 75 per cent and 91 per cent of some 3000 patients treated with *potassium/magnesium aspartate* (1 g of each twice daily) reported pronounced relief from fatigue, while fewer than 25 per cent of people in the control group receiving placebo reported increased energy. Benefits were normally reported within four days although in some cases it took as long as 10 days before benefits were noted. Treatment continued for four to six weeks, and in many instances fatigue did not recur when supplementation stopped. Dryness in the mouth and some gastrointestinal problems were sometimes noted with this treatment.[1]

In an experimental double blind study 87 out of 100 patients suffering from chronic fatigue reported marked improvement after five to six weeks of supplementation with aspartates.[2]

Dr Earl Mindell, author of *The Vitamin Bible*, maintains that aspartic acid increases resistance to fatigue, as well as stamina and endurance. It also detoxifies ammonia from the body, thus enhancing nerve function.[3]

Dr R Krakowitz recommends a full complement (balanced) of free form amino acids to counteract fatigue. Ten to 20 such capsules (containing bet-ween 500 and 800 mg of free form amino acids) are recommended two or three times daily for severe fatigue. This should be between meals with dilut-ed fruit juice and never with a protein (milk for example) as this will delay or stop absorption. This approach should not be used as a long-term strategy but more as a short-term rebuilding approach for people recovering from severe fatigue of whatever cause.[4]

References
[1] Gaby, A. *Aspartic acid and fatigue*, Curr. Nutr. Therapeut., November 1982.
[2] Formica, P. *The Housewife Syndrome*, Current Therapeutic Research, 4:98, 1962.
[3] Mindell, E. Information sheet on L-Aspartic acid, 1981.
[4] Krakowitz, R. *High Energy*, Ballantine Books, New York, 1986.

GALLBLADDER DISEASE

Research into the major nutritional causes of gallbladder disease has shown that a sugar rich diet is a major factor. Sufferers should reduce their intake of fats and of animal based foods, and eat foods rich in fibre (complex carbohydrates). Vegetarians are less likely to suffer from gallbladder disease than non-vegetarians. Women are more prone than men to problems in this area, especially if they are obese and have a high fat and sugar diet. A diet rich in polyunsaturated oils is also harmful: the safest oils are monounsaturated oils such as olive oil. Intolerance to certain foods as well as reduced levels of hydrochloric acid are not uncommonly associated with gallbladder problems. A variety of deficiencies have been noted accompanying gallbladder diseases, including vitamin C and vitamin E, which may beneficially be supplemented, as may essential fatty acids, lecithin and the amino acid taurine (see below).

Animal studies indicate that *taurine* has powerful preventive effects in *gallstone formation*. Three groups of mice were fed a cholesterol-free diet, a diet rich in the elements which help produce gallstones (cholesterol and sodium cholate) and no taurine, or a similar diet with taurine. *Only those mice receiving the gallstone-enhancing diet and no taurine actually developed stones.*[1]

Researchers into the use of taurine on guinea pigs have noted that 'taurine is rapidly emerging as one of the more interesting and ubiquitous amino acids'. Previous studies have shown that the majority of bile acids are joined by either glycine or taurine, making what are in fact natural detergents which increase the emulsification of fats, helping them to be more readily assimilated and easily metabolized. Those which are conjugated (joined) by taurine are the most useful to the bowel. This is influenced by many factors including age, diet, use of drugs, presence of hormones and any disease in the body. In the study in question bile acids were injected into guinea pigs. This would normally be expected to enhance development of gallstones. When *taurine* was given in drinking water up to three days after or five days before the injections, *development of gallstones was prevented*. The conclusion of this study was that an increase in availability of taurine protects against the development of gallstones.[2]

References

[1] Yamanaka, Y. et al. *Effects of dietary taurine on cholesterol gallstone formation*, Journal of Nutritional Science, Vitaminol, 31(2);226–32, 1985.

[2] Dorvil, N. et al. *Taurine prevents cholestasis induced by lithocholic acid sulfate in guinea pigs*, American Journal of Clinical Nutrition, 37(23):221, 1983.

HERPES INFECTION

Since the sexual revolution of the 1960s, herpes has been a major social disease. The discovery some years ago that amino acid manipulation can effectively reduce herpes virus activity and speed healing of active outbreaks has been one of the major phenomena of what Erdmann and Jones call the 'amino revolution'. Herpes attacks (involving HSV 11, or herpes simplex virus type 11) are characterized by the presence of clusters of clear fluid-filled vesicles on the genitalia or face, accompanied by severe pain and itching.

In some cases, there is no more than the occasional 'cold sore', whereas for others the disfigurement and discomfort can lead to major social and sexual problems. In the USA alone, some 300,000 new cases appear each year and roughly a third of the population (some 85 million people) have been exposed to what is known as venereal herpes at some time.

The amino acid strategy is discussed below, but other nutritional aids include zinc and vitamin C (with bioflavonoids) as well as topical application of vitamin E and zinc creams.[1]

The major finding relating to amino acids was that the *herpes virus thrived when there was a high level of arginine* (arginine added to a culture of herpes virus will speed reproduction of the virus) and was *inhibited when there was a high level of lysine*.

Once infected by the herpes virus an individual is unlikely ever to completely get rid of it. The virus remains dormant in the body after the initial infection until it is reactivated as the result of a stress factor such as sunburn, another infection (cold etc), menstruation, emotional upset etc. Stress changes the relative balance of the amino acids arginine and lysine in the circulation and this appears to be a critical factor in the re-emergence of the virus.

Diet also plays a major part so that it is important to choose foods rich in lysine such as meat, potatoes, milk, brewers yeast, fish, chicken, beans and eggs, and to supplement with lysine as well as avoiding arginine rich foods (chocolate, peanuts, nuts, seeds and cereal grains).

It is thought that the reason why these two amino acids are important in herpes infections is because their chemical similarity means that the virus confuses them, incorporating lysine instead of arginine and thus depriving itself of its arginine supplies.[2]

One study showed that *lysine suppressed symptoms of herpes* in 96 per cent of 45 patients tested over a two-year period, with complete remission of herpes outbreaks and no side effects. The researchers reported that 'pain disappeared abruptly overnight in virtually every instance, new vesicles (blisters) failed to appear and resolution in the majority was considered to be more rapid than was their past experience. Patients were infection-free while on lysine, but found that within one to four weeks after stopping lysine, return of lesions could be predicted.' *The amount of lysine required to control herpes varied from case to case but a typical dose to maintain remission was 500 mg daily and active herpes required 1 to 6 g between meals to induce healing.*[3] [4]

A study involving 41 patients indicated that with a daily dose of 1248 mg of lysine hydrochloride herpes outbreaks became less frequent and symptoms less severe. A lower dose of 624 mg failed to achieve this benefit, however.[5] Another study, this time a double blind cross-over trial involving 65 patients, showed that those taking lysine were far freer of recurrences than those taking a placebo.[6]

A combination of lysine and vitamin C together with bioflavonoids is used in the USA to combat the herpes virus, based on the known effects of lysine therapy and studies indicating the other two nutrients to be beneficial. Its brand name is Lysamin-C and each tablet contains 500 mg lysine, 100 mg vitamin C and 100 mg bioflavonoids.[7] [8]

Robert Erdmann PhD has a complex approach to herpes, using lysine as well as a variety of other nutrients including other amino acids. He enhances physical resistance with a combination of tyrosine, DL-phenylalanine, glutamic acid and methionine, together with vitamins B3 and B6, C and magnesium, and mental tranquillity (a major element in recovery from, or control of, herpes infection) with tryptophan, histidine, taurine and glycine.

He adapts the work of the American Dr Emanuel Revici when treating the element of ongoing infection. This involves what are termed *the catabolic amino acids (in this instance) such as methionine, cysteine, taurine, aspartic acid and glutamic acid together with nutrients vitamin A, B6, B12, folic acid, and vitamin C (as calcium ascorbate) and magnesium aspartate, all taken in the evening to coincide with normal body cycles relating to stages of the metabolic process he wishes to influence.* See his book, *The Amino Revolution* (Recommended Reading, page 121).

CAUTION: An animal study on chicks indicated that prolonged use of lysine may stimulate the liver into producing excess levels of cholesterol, and this should be monitored.[9]

References
[1] Warbach, M. *Nutritional Influences on Illness,* Third Line Press, California, 1987.
[2] Passwater, R. *Nutrition and herpes*, Energy Medicine, 1(1):11, 1983.
[3] Kagan, C. *Lysine therapy for herpes simplex,* The Lancet, 1:137(Jan 26 1974)
[4] Griffith, R. et al. *A multicentered study of lysine therapy in herpes simplex infection*, Dermatologica, 156:257–67, 1978.
[5] McCune et al. Cutis, 34:366, 1984.
[6] Milman, N. et. al. *Lysine Prophylaxis in recurrent herpes simplex labialis*, Acta Dermatovener, 60:85–7, 1980.
[7] Beladi, L. *Activity of some flavonoids against viruses*, Annals of the New York Academy of Science.
[8] Leibovitz, B. et al. *Ascorbic acid Neutrophil Function and Immune Response*, International Journal of Nutrition Research, 48:159, 1978.
[9] Schmeisser, D. et al. *Effect of excess dietary lysine may stimulate liver*, Journal of Nutrition, 113(9):1777–83, 1983.

HIGH BLOOD PRESSURE (HYPERTENSION)

High blood pressure is a condition with varying causes, which means that there is no standard desirable treatment. It is the main cause of cardiac disease, which is the major killer in Western society. Anything which can naturally, and without side effects, reduce high blood pressure is of considerable potential value to mankind.

Bad nutrition is a common cause of hypertension as is low stress tolerance and lifestyle factors such as smoking, alcohol, and caffeine consumption (caffeine is found in tea, coffee, coke and chocolate). Nutritionally, a high fibre diet which is low in fat and sugar is the ideal pattern. Vegetarians tend to have lower blood pressure levels than meat eaters. To reduce hypertension, it is important to have a good supply of calcium, magnesium and potassium, and to keep sodium (salt) intake moderate to low.

Specific nutrients such as the essential fatty acids, known as omega-3, and coenzyme Q_{10}, are helpful in reducing hypertension, as is garlic. Stress reduction through relaxation methods or biofeedback techniques are helpful, as is regular exercise.

Amino acids can be useful in the treatment of hypertension in the following ways. For instance, tyrosine may be used, which is a derivative of phenylalanine and a precursor of substances known as catocholamines, a class of neurotransmitter, which includes dopamine and norepinephrine, the presence of both of which are known to decline with age. In studies at Massachusetts General Hospital, psychiatrist Dr Alan Gelenberg administered 100 mg of *tyrosine* three times daily orally for two weeks. He noted that 'The patients showed striking *improvement in mood, self-esteem, sleep, energy level, anxiety and sleep complaints.* No adverse effects were noted.' Plainly this would be an advantage to anyone with anxiety-related hypertension. A dose of tyrosine will result in either an increase in blood pressure in a person in whom it is low, or lowered blood pressure in a person in whom it is high, depending on the activity of certain nerve structures in the brain.[1]

The effectiveness of *tyrosine* in hypertensive individuals may relate to *stress reduction*. Dr Brian Morgan points out that new evidence on animals shows that under extreme stress the brain fails to produce enough norepinephrine to supply the increased demand (and remember its supply declines with age anyway). If animals thus affected were supplied with a high-tyrosine diet, brain levels of norepinephrine (formally known as noradrenaline) rose to adequate levels. *It takes between 50 and 100 mg of tyrosine per kg of body weight in animals to achieve this effect, meaning that a person weighing 100 lb would need 2¼ g daily of tyrosine as a stress reducing brain medication.* This would need to be spread out through the day.[2]

A study in Japan looked at the relationship between taurine and high blood pressure. The taurine content of whole blood and urine was measured in 18 normal and 79 hypertensive patients. Blood levels were found to have no significant differences, but urine showed that normal individuals excreted almost twice the level of taurine as compared to those hypertensives who had what is known as 'essential hypertension', where blood pressure is constantly elevated, perhaps as a result of hardening of the arteries. Those hypertensives with what is known as labile hypertension, which is when there is a rapid rise and fall in blood pressure, excreted roughly the same levels as normal patients. Care was taken to exclude the possibility of any influence of kidney damage in any of the patients. The conclusion was that in high blood pressure the decrease in urinary taurine related to a depression of its formation, rather than to retention.

The results of this study suggested that a deficiency of taurine plays an important role not only in essential hypertension but in the development of atherosclerosis.[3]

Cysteine and methionine both produce taurine, and animal studies indicate that liver dysfunction might have prevented adequate taurine production from cysteine in hypertensive conditions. Other possible influences of taurine on blood pressure may relate to its known effect on heart function, and also on the part it plays in the formation of bile salts, as well as its effect on platelet adhesiveness, discussed in the section on Migraine Headaches (page 96). If taurine is in short supply an increase is noted in certain blood fats (high density lipoproteins) which are harmful to cardiovascular health. Thus there are a number of different ways in which taurine can help high blood pressure and supplementation might be helpful.

References
[1] Philpott, W. *Selective amino acid deficiencies,* Information pamphlet issued by Klaire Laboratories, California.

[2] Morgan B. and R. *Brain Food,* Michael Joseph, London, 1986.

[3] Kohasi, N. *Urinary taurine in essential hypertension,* Japanese Heart Journal, 24(1):91–101, 1983.

IMMUNE FUNCTION ENHANCEMENT, WITH NOTES ON POST VIRAL FATIGUE AND AIDS

There can be few people, in an age when we are all aware of the AIDS crisis, who are unaware of the nature and role of the immune system, the interconnecting and supremely important defence mechanisms which allow us to survive in the face of multiple threats and challenges. Diet plays a fundamental part in the preservation, enhancement and/or restoration of adequate or optimal immune function. Research has clearly shown the ability of nutritional manipulation to affect, modulate and correct the body's immune response.[1]

Space does not permit a review of the many nutritional aids which are available to boost or enhance immune function, since most of the 40 odd vitamins, minerals and trace elements have some effect, and discussion, or even listing, of these would be a lengthy exercise. The amino acids with specific immune enhancing capabilities are discussed below.

For a deeper understanding of the many elements involved in maintaining adequate immune function see Dr Michael Weiner's book *Maximum Immunity* (see Recommended Reading, page 121).

Laboratory studies have shown that carnitine can be used to enhance the response of lymphocytes, the cells which play a major part in the immune system, in both humans and animals.

These were challenged by cancer inducing processes and yet when carnitine was added even in small concentrations, this was shown to be remarkably protective and beneficial.[2]

Deficiencies of amino acids in general, and of specific ones such as taurine and glutamine, are known to weaken the immune response.[3] [4] [5]

A number of amino acids stimulate production by the pituitary gland of a substance known as growth hormone. This has many roles to play in the processes of growth and repair, and also in immune function stimulation. *Arginine (5 to 10 g) and/or ornithine (2½ to 5 g) both stimulate production of growth hormone and can be used to enhance immune function when needed.* These should be taken either individually or together, on an empty stomach at bedtime.

CAUTION: The supplemental use of arginine by schizophrenics is undesirable.[6]

AIDS

Since AIDS is obviously the ultimate example of a compromised immune system, the uses of amino acids in strengthening the immune system generally are a guide to their value in other degenerative conditions.

Here, amino acids are of most value in general health enhancement rather than to obtain specific pharmacological effects (see Chapter 1, page 12), although some specific results are possible, as mentioned above. One of the major symptoms of AIDS is reduction of the body's ability to manufacture adequate protein, accompanied by steady weight loss. As we know, amino acids are the building blocks of protein.

Protein may be inadequately processed by the digestive system for a number of reasons. Thus the food consumed may fail to be reduced to its basic components suitable for absorption and utilization by the body, and if this happens these constituents should be provided in a form which is readily absorbable and usable.

Apart from amino acids with specific therapeutic roles, general free form amino acids (in other words individual, not bound together to make a particular protein) are required. ARC (AIDS related complex) and AIDS patients need this steady supply of amino acids, as almost all of them have impaired digestion and bowel function. The same applies to many chronic diseases, especially those related to what are known as auto-immune diseases (rheumatoid arthritis, lupus) and chronic bowel conditions (colitis etc).

ME

Another group of people has recently been acknowledged as being 'really ill' by medical science, after years of being considered neurotic or hypochondriac. These are the hundreds of thousands of individuals suffering from what is variously known as Post Viral Fatigue Syndrome, Myalgic Encephalomyelitis (ME), Royal Free Disease, Icelandic Disease or 'Closet AIDS', whose major symptom is an overwhelming and profound fatigue after any physical or mental effort.

The condition seems to relate to the ongoing presence of a viral agent (often Epstein-Barr or Cytomegalovirus) which results in a sort of shadow image of AIDS without its more serious, often fatal, implications. What ME and AIDS have in common is a compromised immune system, bowel dysfunction and usually (almost always in fact) Candida overgrowth.

The sort of nutrition desirable for people with ME is the same as that recommended for people with AIDS, and this is outlined below. A variety of nutritional aids as well as herbal and other remedies can help restore ME patients to normal over a period, and the very least that might be done during the recovery stage, apart from the more comprehensive approach described later in this section, would be to take free form amino acids on a regular basis. The dosage should be dependent upon the degree of exhaustion and other factors such as digestive and bowel competence, as well as continuing infections, and can be gradually reduced once energy returns. When the bowel has been damaged or is infested with protozoa and other parasites as well as yeasts such as Candida, as it almost always is in people with ME and AIDS, its permeability may become impaired, allowing absorption of large molecules of partially digested foods which would not happen in normal digestion. This can result in a variety of toxic and allergic reactions.

Amino acid profile

A specialized analysis technique is now available in which various body fluids such as the serum of the blood or urine can be profiled to show the levels of the many amino acids in them. This knowledge is currently backed up by sufficient research to make it possible to compare the findings in any given sample with a standard 'normal' range, thus showing which of the 40 odd amino acids and their metabolites are in excess or deficit, or indeed are within normal ranges. A few companies in the UK and the US work with doctors using nutrition therapy and analyse Candida, AIDS and ARC patients, as well as those with many other serious conditions, during various stages of their illnesses. From the analysis it is possible to obtain a picture of current symptoms as well as to make a prognosis. (For companies that offer this service, see the Resources section on page 120.) There have been major beneficial changes in health and symptomatology as a result of the scientifically applied nutritional supplementation of amino acids which can be formulated after such profiles are completed.

The Tyson organization in the US has records of some 24 individuals with AIDS/ARC who have reversed the negative T-cell ratios and whose health has apparently been restored. At this early stage it is impossible to know their long term prognosis, although there is no reason to anticipate a decline in their regained health. However, the feeling is that it is too early to claim success in dealing with AIDS or ARC, and that such claims can only be made when there are documented records of such individuals surviving in good health for at least three years (the patient with the longest period on this programme currently has been on it for $2\frac{1}{2}$ years).

A formulation of amino acids and associated nutrients suitable for a person with AIDS might include the following (except quantities would depend upon individually assessed needs):

At least half an hour before meals:
- *A balanced amino acid formulation excluding arginine.*
- *A teaspoon of a high potency formulation acidophilus such as Superdophilus or Megadophilus in water.*
- *A teaspoon of Bifido factor (another bacterial culture which repopulates the bowel with 'friendly' bacteria).*
- *If depression is a factor, 1000 to 1500 mg of crystalline L-tyrosine together with 20 mg of vitamin B6 (in its active form of pyridoxal-5'-phosphate) before breakfast and lunch only.*
- *400 to 500 mg of L-tryptophan together with vitamin B6 and vitamin B3 before lunch, evening meal and bedtime.*

During all meals:
- *Two or three high potency formula vitamin/minerals guaranteed from yeast free sources (because of Candida) and including active forms of vitamins B2 and B6. These are best in capsule form as tablets may be indigestible to a person with AIDS or bowel dysfunction.*
- *One or two high potency antioxidant formulations (including Beta carotene, glutathione and corn free vitamin C).*
- *Five to ten high potency amino acid capsules (formulation varies with the needs of the individual and the presence or otherwise of Epstein-Barr virus or herpes infection — see pages 77 and 78 for why patients might need more or less of lysine and/or arginine)*
- *One or more grams of corn free vitamin C.*
- *One high potency, soy free choline supplement including in its formulation phosphatidylcholine (at least 400 mg), phosphatidylinositol (at least 200 mg), phosphatidylethanolamine (400 mg), vitamin B6 (50 mg), methionine (50 mg), serine (50 mg) and manganese (5 mg).*
- *Lysine (500 mg) if herpes is a factor. The effect of lysine on other*

viruses is under investigation and it may be desirable in all viral infections.

- *If herpes infection is not present, 500 to 1000 mg of arginine.*
  After all meals:
- *Half to one teaspoonful Lactobacillus bulgaricus.*

Three meals should be eaten daily.

If Candida is an ongoing problem then the above programme should be modified.

A nutritional programme for a person infected with HIV but not actively with ARC/AIDS conditions would include similar nutrients in highly modified dosages.

These dosages are based on those used by physicians who are treating immune deficiency conditions and Candida with apparent success and are documented in *World Without AIDS* by S. Martin and L. Chaitow.[7]

A different approach is taken by Dr Robert Erdmann. *He proposes use of a supplement which incorporates all the major nutrients known to be involved in immune functions including a number of free form amino acids. This general supplement (formula below) is taken together with supplemented vitamins A (7500iu daily) and C (to bowel tolerance), Beta carotene (the precursor of vitamin A found in vegetables – 15 mg) and essential fatty acids (1500 mg in divided doses) derived from the plant evening primrose.*

The general amino acid supplement contains the following:
arginine 140 mg, ornithine 40 mg, glycine 40 mg, taurine 40 mg, cystine 40 mg, glutamic acid 20 mg, alanine 20 mg, tyrosine 20 mg, tryptophan 20 mg, histidine 20 mg, lysine 20 mg, as well as vitamins B1 20 mg, B2 20 mg, B6 32 mg, B12 200 mcg, vitamin C 40 mg, pantothenic acid 32 mg, folic acid 80 mcg, sorbitol 8 mg, magnesium 40 mg, selenomethionine 20 mcg, zinc gluconate 3.2 mg.

Five capsules containing the above are taken half an hour before breakfast as a general 'health insurance' to maintain immune function.

This intake is increased to three times daily in cases of greater need (AIDS, ME etc). The supplement is marketed in the UK by Nature's Best (see Resources section on page 121) as 'IMU-T'.[8]

The notes given above are meant to give a broad nutritional approach to serious degenerative disease or compromised immune function. Care should also be taken to see that the main diet consists of fresh, wholesome, largely unrefined sources of foods, with a basic low fat, high complex and low simple carbohydrate pattern. Protein intake (from lean meat, game, fish, pulses, nuts and seeds) should also be adequate. An abundance of raw food is suggested, digestion permitting. If not possible then lightly cooked (steamed or stir fried) foods are usually acceptable to a sensitive bowel.

References
1 Corman, L. *Effects of specific nutrients on immune response*, Med. Clin. North America, 69(4):759-91, 1985.
2 Simone, C. et al. *Vitamins and immunity: influence of carnitine on immune system*, Acta Vitaminologica Enzymologica, 4(1-2):135-40, 1982.
3 Stites, D. et al. *Basic and Clinical Immunology*, Lange Medical Publications, pp297-305, 1982.
4 Kafkewitz, D. *Deficiency is immunosupressive*, American Journal of Clinical Nutrition, 37: 1025-30, 1983.
5 Masuda, M. et al. *Influences of taurine*, Japanese Journal of Pharmacology, 34(1):116-18, 1984.
6 Pearson, D. Shaw, S. *Life Extension*, NutriBooks, 1983.
7 Martin, S. Chaitow, L. *World Without AIDS*, Thorsons, 1988.
8 Erdmann, R. AIDS Re-examined, Pamphlet (104) published by Felmore Ltd.

INFERTILITY

There are a number of possible causes of infertility and amino acid therapy can only be effective in some of them. It is worth remembering that most cases of apparent infertility resolve themselves without any treatment and that evidence suggests that as large a proportion of couples attending fertility clinics achieve pregnancy as do apparently infertile couples who do not have any special attention.

In a study in Canada involving 1145 apparently infertile couples, assessed over a period of between two and seven years, pregnancy occurred in 41 per cent (597) of the couples treated by standard medical care, and in 35 per cent of the 548 couples who were untreated. It was also noted that of the pregnancies which took place amongst the treated couples, 31 per cent occurred over three months after the last medical treatment or more than 12 months after surgery. These could then be added to the 'untreated' group, in which case it could be argued that as many as 61 per cent of the pregnancies occurred independent of therapy. This should be of immense satisfaction to the many couples anxious about failure to conceive.[1]

This does not of course mean that nothing can or should be done to establish causes, which at times are simply and easily remedied. A good healthy diet supplemented with vitamin C, zinc and arginine, adequate exercise and rest, abandoning use of tobacco and severely restricting consumption of alcohol, are usually all that is required to prepare the body of the mother for conception.

Organizations such as Foresight (see Resources section on page 122) which advise on preconceptual care of both parents, have statistically proven that such approaches work. This is not to say that in rare cases the heroic methods, pioneered in the UK, of conception achieved outside the womb and reimplanted, are of no value. These however can only be of value to a very limited group of people.[2]

An experimental study was carried out in which 178 men with severely deficient sperm levels and reduced motility of sperm (both major causes of male infertility) were treated with 4 g of arginine a day. Of these 111 achieved marked improvement and 21 others showed moderate improvement. The remaining 25 per cent of patients showed no improvement.[3]

Animal studies would suggest that in cases of infertility there is a deficiency of the amino acid lysine or its derivative carnitine.

Males have very high levels of carnitine in their testes, and higher levels in the bloodstream than females. When animals are deprived of lysine they become infertile due to loss of sperm motility.[4] [5] Changes have also been shown (in various types of infertility) in ornithine, arginine and total amino acid concentrations in the seminal plasma.[6]

Definitive conclusions as to amino acid influence are not yet available but at the least arginine together with zinc and vitamin C should be used by those in need. See also 'Sexual Problems', page 114.

References
[1] New England Journal of Medicine, 309:20, p1201f., 1983.

[2] Warbach, M. *Nutritional Influences on Illness,* Third Line Press, California, 1987.

[3] Schacter, A. et al. *Treatment of oligospermia with Arginine,* Journal of Urology, 110(3):311–13, 1973.

[4] Clinical Chem. Acta, 67:207–12, 1977.

[5] Journal of Nutrition, 107:1209–15, 1977.

[6] Papp, G. et al. *Role of amino acids in fertility,* Int. Urol. Nephrol, 15(2):195–202, 1983.

INFLAMMATION

There are numerous causes of inflammation which should be seen as part of the natural healing process, and should not necessarily be suppressed because of the risk of actually making matters worse. For example, there has recently been a lot of concern in medical circles over the discovery that NSAIDS (non-steroidal anti-inflammatory drugs), used over the past 20 or so years for inflamed joints, have actually worsened the problem. In addition, NSAIDS are also well known for their disastrous effects on digestive and other functions, as witness the anti-arthritic anti-inflammatory drug Opren or the anti-rheumatic drug Butazolidin, now both withdrawn. Thus inflammation should be treated with caution and simple methods such as cold compresses or ice applications are often far safer and more effective than medication.

Sometimes however treatment is needed and here again nutrients have shown themselves to be useful, for example vitamin C, vitamin E, zinc, omega-3 and -6 fatty acids, bioflavonoids such as quercetin, proteolytic enzymes such as bromelain (from pineapple plant), alone or in combination. Certain amino acids have also been found to be useful including creatine, phenylalanine and tryptophan (D and L forms) and valine (also D and L). Both phenylalanine and tryptophan have also been shown to have powerful analgesic (pain relieving) properties, as we shall see in the section on Pain Control (see page 102).

In animal studies it was shown that creatine was as effective an anti-inflammatory medicine as was the drug phenylbutazone in both chronic and acute situations, whilst producing no gastro-intestinal reactions. It was also noted for its pain killing (analgesic) effects.[1]

It has been suggested that D-phenylalanine is capable of reducing inflammation in much the same way as it reduces pain, because of its ability to slow down the natural breakdown of pain killing substances (endorphins and encephalins) produced by the brain and allow them to maintain their role for longer. That inflammation would be reduced in joints in much the same manner is supported by animal studies, for when such endorphins were injected into rat paws inflammatory processes were neutralized.[2][3]

Tryptophan acts in a similar manner to phenylalanine. A study on animals found that tryptophan (L or DL) was as effective as phenylbutazone in suppressing acute or chronic inflammatory responses but not in exactly the same way. Similar studies using valine were assessed by the same researchers, with good results.[4]

For suggestions on dosage, follow the advice given in the section on Pain Control on pages 102-4.

References

[1] Khanna, N. et al. *Anti-inflammatory activity in creatine,* Arch. Int. Pharmacodyn Ther., 231(2):340-50, 1978.

[2] Millinger, G. S. *Neutral amino acid therapy for management of chronic pain* Cranio 4(2):156-63, 1986.

[3] Ferreira, S. et al. *Prostaglandin hyperalgesia: The opiod antagonists,* Prostaglandins, 18:181-200, 1979.

[4] Madan, B. et al. *Anti-inflammatory activity of L and DL tryptophan,* Indian Journal of Medical Research, 68:708-13, 1978 and *Anti-inflammatory activity of DL-valine,* Indian Journal of Experimental Biology 16:834-6, 1978.

INSOMNIA

One of the major successes of amino acid therapy has been related to sleep disturbances. Drs Goldberg and Kaufman, in their book *Natural Sleep*, describe the research on tryptophan and sleep carried out by Dr Ernest Hartman of Boston State Hospital. In a series of 11 experiments conducted over a period of seven years up to 1978 Dr Hartman documented the effects of tryptophan on both animal and human subjects. All the studies compared tryptophan, at various doses, with placebo substances under double blind conditions. Tryptophan and the placebo were administered in 1 g dosage 20 minutes before bedtime, and a variety of physiological variables were recorded including changes in brainwave pattern. Those tested included both normal sleepers and insomniacs.

The findings showed a speeding up, by 50 per cent, of what is called sleep latency (the time it takes to go to sleep), and a deeper, more refreshing sleep experienced as a rule. No side effects were noted.[1]

Hartman's report on tryptophan showed the following:
1. Increased sleep latency.
2. Doses lower than 1 g were not effective and larger doses did not make for more improvement in sleep patterns. 1 g is the dose recommended for most insomniacs although those with severe sleep problems may benefit from higher intakes.
3. Continued use usually helped those not initially showing signs of benefit.
4. If doses were kept below 15 g daily, no side effects were noted of any consequence.[2]

Research into how tryptophan works involved the administration of between 1 and 4 g before bedtime in ten male patients, all chronic insomniacs, aged between 30 and 72. There was a 30 per cent sustained relief from insomnia, with no side effects, in 90 per cent of the patients. It is thought that the formation of the calming neurotransmitter serotonin (from tryptophan) is its means of action.[3]

A double blind, cross-over study, involving 20 males, was carried out to assess the effects of a single dose of tryptophan or tyrosine, against a matched placebo. Various tests of mood state were performed. The results showed that tryptophan increased the feelings of tiredness and decreased feelings of vigour and alertness, although this was mostly imagined by the subjects with no objective evidence. Tyrosine, by contrast, was found to increase alertness and reaction times. The conclusions were that tryptophan had significant sedative properties and that, despite the feelings it created, it did not, unlike drugs, impair performance of normal tasks such as driving a car.[4]

Goldberg and Kaufman remind us that vitamin B6 is essential for the body to use tryptophan efficiently. Dosage of 50 to 150 mg is suggested.

Tryptophan is more efficiently utilized if taken with a small amount of carbohydrate (half a biscuit for example) 20 minutes before retiring. Avoidance of caffeine, low intake of alcohol and adequate exercise and relaxation are also desirable for better sleep.

A nutritional 'sleeping tablet' combining tryptophan, vitamin B6 and two other factors, calcium and magnesium, is marketed as *Somnamin* by Larkhall Laboratories (see Resources section on page 121).

References:
[1] Goldberg, P. Kaufman, D. *Natural Sleep,* Rodale Press, 1978.
[2] Hartman, L. *Report to an American Medical Association symposium,* reported in Clinical Psychiatry News, March 1985.
[3] Fitten, L. et al. *Tryptophan as hypnotic in special patients,* Journal of the American Geriatric Society, 33:294–7, 1985.
[4] Leiberman, H. et al. *Effects of dietary neurotransmitters on human behaviour,* American Journal of Clinical Nutrition, 42(2):36–70.

MENOPAUSAL PROBLEMS

There are many different symptoms experienced by women at the change of life. The more obvious and common ones, though, are depression (see page 63), fatigue (see page 73), and hot flashes. Hot flashes and sweats can be helped by supplementation of bioflavonoids and vitamin E.[1] Tryptophan has also been shown to be useful in such cases since its deficiency may relate to menopausal depression. Low blood and oestrogen levels were found in women with this problem.[2]

In another study, methionine was found to be handled differently by pre- and postmenopausal women. The role of sulphur (which is part of methionine) was observed in ten premenopausal and ten postmenopausal women, all of whom were in good health, and the results compared with two groups of ten men of comparable ages. After overnight fasting each person tested was given 0.1 g of methionine per kg of their body weight. The blood was tested immediately before and eight hours after this 'loading' test for methionine derivatives including methionine itself, homocystine, cystine, and homocysteine-cysteine.

In the fasting state, before supplementation, premenopausal women and both groups of men showed similar levels of all substances tested for, while postmenopausal women had low values of the same substances.

They also displayed excessive levels of homocysteine after the loading test, showing that before the menopause women can metabolize methionine and its derivatives more efficiently. This extra efficiency in younger women is thought to account, at least in part, for their lower incidence of cardiovascular disease during childbearing years.

Menopausal women should be careful in the degree of methionine supplementation they undertake.[3]

References
[1] Werbach, M. *Nutritional Influences on Illness,* Third Line Press, California, 1987.
[2] Editorial in the British Medical Journal, 1:242–3, 1976.
[3] Journal of Clinical Investigation, 72(6):1971–6.

MIGRAINE HEADACHES

Migraine headaches have a number of causes, both emotional and physical.

Food sensitivities also play an important part. One study identified colouring and flavouring agents in food, alcohol, chocolate, coffee, tea, foods containing tyramine, as well as certain vitamins and minerals and foods contaminated with pesticides, as all causing headaches in sensitive individuals.[1]

In particular, the food substances which contain elements that lead to migraine in sensitive individuals include:

Nitrites found in cured and luncheon meats in large amounts. Thus bacon, sausages, ham, salami, hot dogs etc are possible foods to eliminate.

Monosodium glutamate found in Chinese cooking (restaurant food that is) and much canned food. Even normally non-headache subjects will develop a thumping skull when this food additive (the sticky glutinous stuff so obvious in much Chinese restaurant food) is present in large amounts, leading to the well known medical condition, Chinese Restaurant Syndrome.

Tyramine found in milk, cheese, especially mature varieties, chocolate, eggs, wheat, peanuts, citrus fruits, tomatoes, pork, pickled herrings, salted dried fish, sausages, chicken liver, beef, Italian broad beans (fava), sauerkraut, vanilla, yeast and yeast extracts, soy sauce, beer, ale, red wine, Sauternes, Riesling wines, champagne, sherry, port, and in fact in alcohol of all sorts.[2]

An experimental double blind study found that 93 per cent of 88 children with severe and frequent migraines recovered when placed on a special diet (known as an oligoantigenic diet) which eliminated foods that caused the problem. Once identified, the foods were used again, provoking headaches and thus proving the connection. The foods most suspect were dairy produce, eggs, chocolate, wheat and some meats (pork).[3]

It is believed that the actual mechanism causing the headache involves an abnormality in the function of blood platelets, allowing for increased concentration, reduced circulatory efficiency and the specific symptoms of migraine headaches. A study was conducted into the connection between *taurine* and platelet adhesiveness. Taurine is a sulphur containing amino acid and it was noted that during migraine attacks, taurine platelet levels were significantly greater than in the period of five to ten days following the headache. The researchers noted that more than one chemical species was involved in these changes apart from taurine, including serotonin (derived from tryptophan).

The significance of these findings is not clear although it would suggest that manipulation of taurine and tryptophan levels could possibly reduce migraine incidence.[4]

Erdmann and Jones suggest use of *DLPA* (see section on Pain Control, page 102) for treatment of migraine, as well as *tryptophan*, stating that its ability to help in this respect can 'be attributed to its serotonin-producing pathway and the dilatory effect it has on blood vessels – relieving the pressure areas which cause migraine by distributing the blood more widely.'[5]

Ironically, although deficiency of serotonin (which is a derivative of tryptophan) is a cause of migraine, so are excess levels of serotonin. It has been pointed out that headaches (along with fatigue and many other symptoms) increase in an atmosphere of positive ionization. This is the sort of atmospheric electrical change which occurs when a storm is coming up, or there is a strong prevailing wind, such as a mistral, or the sort of atmosphere found in centrally heated, air conditioned, or smoke polluted modern offices and apartments. It seems that production of serotonin is stimulated by this alteration in positive air ion content and that this can be effectively reversed by the simple use of a negative ionizer. These instruments are now readily available and are fairly inexpensive.[6] [7]

The use of the herb feverfew reduces platelet aggregation, thus effectively inhibiting migraine attacks.[8]

References
[1] Cephalgia, 2(2):111–24, 1982.
[2] Harold Gelb, *Killing Pain Without Prescription,* Harper and Row, 1980.
[3] Egger, J. et al. *Is migraine a food allergic disease?* The Lancet, pp865–9, Oct 15 1983.
[4] Dhopesh, V. et al. *Change in Platelet taurine and migraine,* Headache Journal, 22(4):165, 1982.
[5] Erdmann, R. Jones, M. *The Amino Revolution,* Century, 1987.
[6] Soyka, F. *The Ion Effect,* Dutton, New York, 1977.
[7] Mann, J. *Secrets of Life Extension,* Harbor Publishing Co., 1980.
[8] Johnson, E. et al. *Efficacy of Feverfew in treatment of migraine,* British Medical Journal, 291:569–73, 1985.

MULTIPLE SCLEROSIS

Supplementation and dietary manipulation have in many instances allowed a remission of MS symptoms. Those most investigated include the essential fatty acids derived from oil of evening primrose. Injections of thiamine have also been found useful, and deficiencies of calcium, vitamin D and pyridoxine may also be causes. Massive supplementation of B vitamins, vitamin C and many other nutrients including the amino acid phenylalanine have been reported as helpful, as has removal of dental amalgams which may be producing mercury toxicity (these should be replaced with composite dental materials including ceramic type substances). A high fat diet interferes with the production of derivatives of essential fatty acids and therefore a low fat diet is considered desirable.

The amino acid phenylalanine has been reported to be useful.[1]

In an experimental double blind trial 50 MS patients were treated with D-phenylalanine and electrical stimulation (TENS). Forty-nine of the 50 showed improvements such as better bladder control, greater mobility and less depression.[2]

Use of amino acids such as cysteine and glutathione (along with zinc, calcium and vitamin C) may assist in elimination of the toxic heavy metal mercury, which produces symptoms similar to MS, from the body.

References
[1] Werbach, M. *Nutritional Influences on Illness,* Third Line Press, California, 1987.
[2] Winter, A. *New Treatment for MS,* Neurological & Orthopaedic Journal of Medicine & Surgery, 5(1), April 1984.

OVERWEIGHT PROBLEMS

In the main, weight problems are caused by the problem of eating too much of the wrong foods and getting inadequate exercise. Supplementation with vitamin C, evening primrose oil and coenzyme Q_{10} can assist in recovery but cannot be a substitute for correct eating and exercise. The diet should reduce, or avoid, refined carbohydrates (especially sugar) and replace these with high fibre foods and complex carbohydrates, with much of the food eaten raw. Calorie control is one aspect of reducing weight and this calls for a steady application of basic rules rather than sudden heroic efforts.

Brilliant research has shown that there are a number of ways in which amino acids can be used to help control appetite and select desirable foods at mealtime. *It may be possible to reduce a desire for sugary foods by supplementation with glutamine, which is known to be a good way of reducing alcohol craving. Dosage is between 200 mg and 1 g three times daily.*[1] [2] [3]

In one study, healthy young male volunteers of normal body weight were given a standard breakfast. They were then given either a capsule of *tryptophan* or a placebo 45 minutes before a buffet style (self service) lunch. Those who had taken the tryptophan selected food of significantly fewer calories than those who had taken the placebo. In another similar study consisting of 15 people the same *more desirable selection of food* was noted when 2 g or 3 g of tryptophan were given, but not when only 1 g was supplemented.

The most noticeable difference was that those receiving adequate tryptophan chose fewer bread rolls and biscuits and reported that they were not as hungry as usual.[4]

Tryptophan was also the subject of a study of 62 overweight Swiss patients, when it was used in combination with what is known as a protein-sparing modified fast (PSMF). These people were questioned as to the times when they usually experienced cravings for carbohydrates. They were asked to drink a liquid which contained either tryptophan or a placebo twice daily for three months, at times of 30 or 60 minutes before the expected craving, or at least 60 minutes after a meal. The trial was double blind in that neither the doctors nor the patients knew who was consuming tryptophan. At the start of the study all the patients were at least 40 per cent over their normal body weight. Those receiving tryptophan increased their weight loss by 3.4 kg in the first month and 2.6 kg in each of the next two months.

The best results were noted in those who were not grossly overweight at the outset.[5]

Another study was carried out on people of normal weight, and people who were slightly and very overweight, in which a combination of amino acids (*phenylalanine 3 g, valine 2 g, methionine 2 g, tryptophan 1 g)* or a placebo was given half an hour before a meal. Between 8 and 32 g of the amino acid mixture was given. *A significantly reduced intake of food was noted* in those who were above their body weight, but not in those of normal weight. This may have been the result of stimulation of the gastrointestinal hormone cholecystokinin, which is thought to have the effect of reporting to the brain that enough has been eaten to satisfy needs.

Previous studies have shown that phenylalanine has the effect of stimulating production of cholecystokinin.

It is also known that tryptophan has the same effect as a carbohydrate meal, causing the release of the neurotransmitter serotonin in the brain, which could explain the lower selection of carbohydrate foods in overweight people who have had tryptophan supplemented.[6]

Animals allowed to choose between carbohydrate and protein rich foods not only regulate the amount of calories consumed, but also the proportion of protein and carbohydrate. Many overweight people, on the other hand, consume half their daily intake of calories in the form of carbohydrate-rich snacks, often associated with a strong craving. This may be the result of an abnormality in the brain's serotonin release process, which tryptophan can moderate.[7]

The strategy to adopt would appear to be to eat a small amount of carbohydrate together with a gram or two of tryptophan (but not if you are pregnant) about 20 minutes before a meal. This causes release of serotonin and ensures that less carbohydrate and more protein will be eaten, and that the food chosen will be more appropriate to weight loss.

For overall lowering of appetite take 700 to 1100 mg of phenylalanine to induce release of cholycystokinin within half an hour. Glutamine supplementation as discussed above will reduce sugar craving.[8]

References

1 Passwater, R. *Glutamine: the surprising brain fuel,* Educational pamphlet.
2 Goodwin, F. National Institute for Mental Health, quoted in APA Psychiatric News, Dec. 5 1986.
3 Williams R. *Nutrition Against Disease,* Bantam Books, 1981.
4 Heboticky, N. *Effects of L tryptophan on short term food intake,* Nutritional Research, 5(6):595–607, 1985.
5 Heraif, E. et al. International Journal of Eating Disorders, 4(3):281–92.
6 Butler R. et al. American Journal of Clinical Nutrition, 34(10): 2045, 1982.
7 Wurtman, R. *Behavioural effects of nutrients,* The Lancet, p1145, May 21 1983.
8 Chaitow, L. *Amino Acids in Therapy,* Thorsons, 1985 and *Slimming and Health Workbook,* Thorsons, 1989.

PAIN CONTROL

Phenylalanine and tryptophan are the two key elements in pain control (as they are in weight control and depression). Pain should be thought of as a clear warning from the body that all is not well. Thus simply obliterating pain, whether with medication or other means of pain control such as acupuncture or electrical stimulation (TENS), without consideration as to what the alarm indicates, is poor medicine.

However, once the cause is attended to it is clearly desirable to control or reduce the level of pain. Acupuncture and acupressure techniques achieve much of their effectiveness, it is thought, via stimulation of the release of natural self-produced pain killers. These are known variously as endorphins and encephalins. It is thought that phenylalanine enhances pain relief by slowing down the breakdown of these body-produced pain relievers, giving them a longer time to act. The psychological element is also very important in pain relief: the more anxious we are, the greater we perceive the pain; the more relaxed we are, the less we perceive the pain. The same degree of pain will at different times be perceived as greater or lesser according to whether we are tense and anxious or calm and relaxed. Tryptophan and phenylalanine have both been shown to have relaxing and calming actions (see Depression, page 63). Thus these versatile fractions of protein have a dual purpose: in calming and in pain control.

An experimental study was conducted in which 43 patients, mainly with *osteoarthritis*, were given 250 mg *D-Phenylalanine (DPA)*, three to four times daily, for between four and five weeks. During the last two weeks, *significant pain relief* was noted, especially in those patients with osteoarthritis. The DPA became more effective as pain decreased.[1]

In an experimental double blind cross-over study it was found that after two weeks of taking 250 mg of *DPA* three times a day, seven out of 21 chronic pain patients were able to *stop all other medication* and to note a *50 per cent reduction in pain levels*. Of those patients on a placebo only one improved while 13 patients showed no significant improvement from either DPA or placebo.[2]

Studies showed that in animal experiments previously unsuccessful acupuncture became more effective once *phenylalanine* had been supplemented, and that the effects of *pain relief* were more persistent. Similar results were obtained in humans. Administration of *phenylalanine* (2000 mg) one hour before a dental procedure resulted in an *increased threshold of pain*, which further rose after an acupuncture treatment. Pre-administration of DPA enhanced the analgesic (pain relieving) effects of humans undergoing acupuncture for low back and dental surgery, where acupuncture alone was ineffective. [3] [4]

A study was conducted involving 14 cancer patients to see the effects of injection of 3 mg of endorphins (the natural pain killers of the body which DPA protects from degradation, which cannot be taken by mouth as they are destroyed in the stomach). All the patients had chronic, sleep preventing pain which had resisted powerful narcotic medication, yet after this treatment they all reported profound and longlasting *complete* relief from their pain which took about five minutes to appear and which lasted for a day and a half. There were no side effects (apart from some of the patients becoming extremely happy!).

A similar study involved women who were about to deliver their babies. They were given just 1 mg of beta-endorphin by injection and all labour pains disappeared completely, with no side effects, apart from mild drowsiness. The relief of all pain was noted for between 12 and 32 hours. It is considered that many chronic pain sufferers and people with low pain thresholds have a low level of natural endorphins. In some studies the levels have been nearly 90 per cent lower than those in people with normal tolerance to pain. DLPA retards the breakdown of endorphins and thus ensures longer natural pain relief. [5] [6]

Tryptophan, in doses of 2 to 4 g daily, taken with sugar and with no protein for 90 minutes before and after taking, had *pain relieving effects*. Thirty chronic pain patients were involved in a double blind study in which they were placed on a high carbohydrate, low fat, low protein diet and were randomly assigned to receive 3 g of tryptophan or a placebo.

After four weeks pain thresholds had risen in the tryptophan group but not the placebo group. [7]

In an experimental double blind study involving 30 normal individuals, some received 2 g of *tryptophan* daily in divided doses and others a placebo. After eight days, dental-pulp stimulation was performed to assess levels of pain tolerance. This was much higher (that is *higher tolerance and therefore less pain noted*) in those receiving tryptophan. There were side effects of itching, nausea, weight loss and mood elevation in the tryptophan group.[8]

The form most generally available of phenylalanine is a combination of the D and L forms. This is because of the great expense of the D form alone.

The following dosage of DLPA is suggested:

Two tablets of 375 mg 20 minutes before meals three times daily. If after three weeks there has not been a considerable relief of chronic pain then the dose should be doubled. If there is still no relief then DLPA should be abandoned. There is a small percentage of failure (five to 15 per cent). Relief is usually noted within seven days at which time supplementation should be stopped until pain returns.[9]

References

[1] Balagot, R. Advances in Pain Research and Therapy, 5:289–92, 1983.

[2] Budd, K. *Use of DPA and enkephalinase inhibitor in treatment of intractable pain,* Advances in Pain Research and Therapy, 5:305–8, 1983.

[3] Takishige, M. Advances in Pain Research and Therapy, 563–8, 1983

[4] Mesayoshi, H. *Analgesic effect induced by phenylalanine during acupuncture analgesia in humans,* Advances in Pain Research and Therapy, 577–82, 1983.

[5] Oyama, T. et al. *Intrathecal use of beta-endorphin as a powerful analgesic in man,* Advances in Pharmacology and Therapeutics, 11:39–43, 1981.

[6] Fox, A. and B. *DLPA,* Thorsons, 1987.

[7] Seltzer, S. et al. *Effects of dietary tryptophan on chronic maxillofacial pain,* Journal of Psychiatric Research, 17:181–6, 1982–3.

[8] Seltzer, S. *Alternation of Human Pain Threshold,* Pain, 13(4):385–93, 1982.

[9] Chaitow, L. *Amino Acids in Therapy,* Thorsons, 1985.

PARKINSON'S DISEASE

This condition is characterized by inability to control movement, leading to tremors, loss of use of the hands and arms, and in the worst cases, of speech. Treatment using L-Dopa is currently the favoured approach. This is not effective in all cases and in any case becomes less powerful in time. A *low protein diet* during the day increases sensitivity to L-Dopa, allowing it to be more effective in lower dosages.

Methionine has been shown to improve symptoms of patients already deriving benefits from standard medical care. In one study, 15 patients received 1 g a day of methionine, which was gradually increased to 5 g a day, without interruption of normal medication.

After two months, ten patients showed improvements with regard to activity level, ease of movement, mood, sleep, attention span, muscular strength, concentration, and speech, and walking became less difficult. Symptoms such as drooling and trembling did not improve in all cases. There were two cases in which side-effects of either diarrhoea or nausea were noted.[1]

Another study examined the use of *phenylalanine (DPA)*. Fifteen patients received 250 mg twice daily. After four weeks neurological examination revealed significant improvements in the degree of rigidity, walking disabilities, speech problems and depression. There was no improvement in the tremor.[2]

Patients receiving L-Dopa may become deficient in tryptophan, because of competition for uptake between these two substances, and certain symptoms such as depression may appear as a result.[3]

One study, commenting on the low level of tryptophan in Parkinson patients, showed a considerable improvement in mental symptoms, when intravenous and oral supplementation was introduced. This suggests that a precautionary addition of tryptophan or protein should be given to people taking L-Dopa.[4]

In another study, 40 patients received either L-Dopa and tryptophan or L-Dopa and a placebo. The L-Dopa produced benefits in terms of reduced tremor, rigidity, walking difficulties, posture etc in both groups while a significant improvement was seen in the ability to perform certain tasks in the group also receiving tryptophan. Only this group showed an improvement in their mood and drive.[5]

It is not suggested that anyone with Parkinson's disease should experiment with amino acids on their own but that they might draw the attention of their medical advisers to the possibility of enhancing their current medication in this manner.

References
[1] Smythies, J. *Treatment of Parkinson's disease with methionine*, Southern Medical Journal, 77(12):1577, 1984.
[2] Heller, B. et al. *Therapeutic action of D-phenylalanine in Parkinson's disease*, Arzneim-Forsch, 26:577-9, 1976.
[3] *Levodopa and depression in Parkinsonism*, The Lancet, 1:140, 1971.
[4] Lehmann, J. *Tryptophan malabsorption in levodopa treated patients*, Acta Medica Scandinavia, 194:181-9, 1973.
[5] Coppen, A. et al. *Levodopa and L-tryptophan therapy in Parkinsonism*, The Lancet, 1:654-7, 1972.

PEPTIC ULCER

Surgery is often used to deal with peptic ulcers which fail to heal under normal medical care. A number of lifestyle and dietary strategies may assist, including avoidance of smoking, milk, alcohol, sugary and spicy foods. Nutrients such as bioflavonoids, vitamin B6, vitamin A, E, and C, as well as zinc and the amino acid glutamine, may also help.[1]

An experimental double blind trial on peptic ulcer patients involved standard treatment and either glutamine (400 mg four times daily one hour before meals and before retiring) or lactose. After four weeks all seven of the patients receiving glutamine had healed, compared with seven out of 14 receiving lactose.[2]

References
[1] Werbach, M. *Nutritional Influences on Illness,* Thorsons, 1989.
[2] Shive, W. et al. *Glutamine in treatment of peptic ulcer,* Texas State Journal of Medicine, pp840-3, November 1957.

PREMENSTRUAL SYNDROME (PMS)

The work of Dr G Abraham in California has identified four basic patterns of PMS (or premenstrual tension, PMT).[1] These are:

1. PMT (A) which has as its main features anxiety (hence the (A) in the title) and also mood swings, irritability, insomnia and nervous tension.
2. PMT (D) which has depression as its main feature (D) together with forgetfulness, crying and confusion.
3. PMT (C) with craving (C) for sweet foods as its main symptom, along with headache, increased appetite, palpitations, dizziness and extreme tiredness.
4. PMT(H) which relates to retention of fluid (H for hyperhydration) involving rapid weight gain (over 3 lbs) before the menstrual cycle, swelling of extremities, tender breasts and abdominal bloating.

Various nutrients can assist in all these types of PMS: magnesium, evening primrose oil, vitamin B6, and vitamin E. Reduction of intake of salt and sugar, dairy foods and calcium, and avoidance of caffeine, nicotine and alcohol also help.

Arnold Fox advises taking amino acids in combination with other nutrients. He suggests taking 500 mg of tryptophan after breakfast and dinner, if necessary increasing this to six capsules daily, three in the morning and three in the evening (remember that this is suggested as a part of a comprehensive programme, together with vitamins B, C, E, magnesium, zinc, evening primrose oil etc at various times of the day).

He further suggests that DLPA (D and L phenylalanine) be taken as follows. If weight is more than 110lbs, he suggests 375 mg with breakfast and lunch. If no result is forthcoming he increases this to include 375 mg with dinner. This is done for four to seven days before PMS symptoms usually appear in the cycle, stopping at the end of the menstrual flow.[2]

(See Resources section, page 122, for address of PMT advisory centre).

References

[1] Abraham, G. *Premenstrual tension problems*, Obstetrics and Gynaecology 3(12):1–39, 1980.
[2] Fox, A. and B. *DLPA*, Long Shadow Books, 1985.

PROTECTION OF CELLS FROM TOXICITY AND RADIATION

Over the past few years there has been increasing evidence as to the ways in which certain nutrients can offer protection to cells when these are exposed to what could be dangerous levels of toxic materials or radiation.

Dr I Brekhman reports from the Soviet Union that as part of the country's space programme over 25,000 different chemical substances have been analysed and examined in order to discover effective protective substances against the effects of radiation. The two amino acids which are now incorporated into the 'cocktail' of nutrients given to cosmonauts are histidine (1 to 2 g per day) and tryptophan (for relaxation, not radiation protection).[1]

Radiation damage occurs in large part due to release of what are called free radicals. These electrically charged entities are capable of causing cellular damage on a large scale. The normal body defence against these includes glutathione peroxidase, which is itself dependent upon selenium and the amino acid cysteine (as well as glutamic acid and glycine). Cysteine is itself a powerful antioxidant (destroyer of dangerous free radicals) and when combined with vitamin C and B1 it has a protective effect on cells exposed to radiation.

During periods of exposure to radiation of any sort a dosage of 1 to 3 g daily of cysteine, and 1 or 2 g of glutathione, taken away from mealtimes in divided doses with diluted fruit juice, is suggested.[2]

NOTE: Diabetics should not take cysteine without guidance, and manic depressives should not take histidine.

In an attempt to assess the protective function of a variety of nutrients, human cells (lymphoblasts) were cultured and then exposed to toxic substances. The presence on their own of the amino acid taurine and the mineral zinc protected cells from retinol-induced damage, and when these nutrients were used together they abolished the swelling and enhanced cell function by 55 per cent. Vitamin E was also effective in protecting cells in this way. When the three substances were used together, they afforded *complete* protection.

It should be noted that we lose taurine under certain conditions, including myocardial infarction, skeletal damage, physical and emotional stress, high alcohol consumption, and deficiency in zinc.[3]

One of the most toxic compounds known is carbon tetrachloride which can cause massive damage to the liver. The amino acids aspartic acid, methionine and tyrosine were found to protect against liver damage in animals when given 30 minutes before exposure to the toxin. Aspartic acid, tyrosine and cystine also offered protection when given up to six hours after exposure. The toxin was still present in the liver but the tissues were protected.[4]

Glutathione and cystine protect tissues against the ill effects of tobacco smoke and of alcohol; however, they should not be regarded as antidotes to smoking and excessive drinking.

References
[1] Brekhman, I. *Man and Biologically Active Substances*, Pergamon Press, 1980.
[2] Saksonov, P. Antiradiation Protection (in Foundations of Space Biology and Medicine), pp317–47, Nauka Moscow, 1975.
[3] Pasantes, M. et al. *Protective effect of taurine, zinc and tocopherol on retinol in-duced damage to human lymphoblasts,* Journal of Nutrition, 114(12): 2256–61.
[4] British Journal of Experimental Pathology, 64(2);166–71, 1983.

RESTLESS LEG SYNDROME

This condition may relate to folic acid deficiency and is often improved if folic acid and vitamin E are supplemented and caffeine containing substances are avoided.

The condition is often accompanied by (or accompanies) depression and other health problems, and can be of a severe nature, not allowing the sufferer any peace, with a constant need for the leg to 'jump' and to move around. Symptoms are often worse at night.

Tryptophan has been found useful in treating cases of restless leg syndrome. One elderly gentleman, who suffered from very high blood pressure and kidney failure (he had for several years been having dialysis), had also been having for the past three years symptoms of crawling, tingling and burning sensations in his legs, especially in the evenings and when resting during the day, resulting in insomnia and depression. No neurological causes were found for the symptoms and various drugs proved ineffective. One gram of L-tryptophan twice daily cleared both the symptoms affecting the legs and the insomnia within three days, with no side effects.

In another case an elderly man with chronic obstructive lung disease, who was receiving steroid (cortisone) type medication, had a two-year history of restless leg syndrome, with resultant depression and insomnia. Medication was ineffective, but when he was given 2 g of L-tryptophan at night this produced dramatic relief of both the insomnia and the restless leg symptoms, within four nights, with no side effects.[1]

References
[1] Sandyk, R. L-tryptophan in treatment of restless leg syndrome. Letter to the American Journal of Psychiatry, 143(4):554–5, 1986.

RHEUMATOID ARTHRITIS

This is a severe and often crippling disease which is not fully understood. In many instances nutritional manipulation may help, including a diet low in fats and one that excludes food from animal sources (a vegan diet). Care should be taken to ensure optimal levels of nutrient intake.

Several nutrients have been found helpful including vitamin C, vitamin B5 (pantothenic acid), selenium, zinc, and sulphur. Particular food sensitivities may be a factor in rheumatoid arthritis and supplementation of omega 3 and 6 fatty acids as well as various nutrients such as bromelain and quercetin have been reported to give symptomatic relief.

Amino acids are useful in a number of ways. For instance, it has been found that levels of histidine are very low in rheumatoid arthritis patients although other amino acids are in normal supply.[1][2] Supplementation with histidine has been found helpful, although not dramatically so. In an experimental double blind study patients were treated with either $4\frac{1}{2}$ g histidine daily or a placebo. After 30 weeks there was a biochemical change showing benefits for those patients receiving histidine and there was some evidence of improvement in those patients with a long duration of the disease.[3]

Phenylalanine (see dosages in Pain Control section) is reported to have dramatically reduced symptoms in a 47-year-old female patient with rheumatoid arthritis.[4]

Tryptophan has been effective in reducing swelling in animals with rheumatoid arthritis .[5]

References
[1] Journal of Clinical Investigation, 55:1164, 1977.
[2] Journal of Chronic Disease, 30:115, 1977.
[3] Pinals, R. et al. *Treatment of RA with L-histidine*, Journal of Rheumatology, 4(4):414–19, 1977.
[4] Anabolism 4 (2),1985.
[5] Journal of the American Podiatry Association, 70(2):65, 1980.

SCHIZOPHRENIA

This major mental illness has been found to have at least two distinct forms, one with a very high degree of histamine in the brain and one with a very low level. These two groups together account for fully two thirds of all schizophrenic individuals.

The high histamine schizophrenic are called histadelics. These are usually suicidally depressed. Methionine may be used to decrease levels of histamine (see section on Sexual Problems, page 114) since it detoxifies the body of excess levels. In addition to methionine, Pfeiffer and Iliev, the main researchers into this application of amino acid therapy, suggest using magnesium, zinc and calcium lactate.

Those schizophrenics with very low levels of histamine are known as histapenics, and supplementation of histidine can result in balancing this deficiency. Pfeiffer believes that histamine is a neurotransmitter for some as yet unidentified region of the brain.

As noted in the section on Behaviour Modification (page 56), aggressive behaviour in schizophrenics was modified by supplementation of tryptophan in a double blind cross-over study.[1]

Naturally in a condition as serious as schizophrenia such supplementation should be directed by an expert who can monitor the progress of the individual. This is not a suitable condition for self-medication.[2]

References
[1] Morand, C. et al. Biological Psychiatry, 18:575–8, 1983.
[2] Pfeiffer, C. *Mental and Elemental Nutrients*, Keats Publishers, New Canaan, 1975.

SEXUAL PROBLEMS

We have already examined the role of arginine in infertility (page 89). This section relates more to frigidity and impotence, as well as to a failure to experience orgasm and premature ejaculation.

The experience of sexual arousal involves histamine release, as does the experience of an orgasm itself. If histidine levels are low, histamine production will be reduced, leading to frigidity in women, and failure of orgasm in both sexes. Histidine is therefore crucial in helping people with this problem.

Major research into this subject was conducted by Dr Carl Pfeiffer who established that *additional histidine given to frigid women in doses of 500 mg before each meal three times daily resulted in a restoration of enjoyment of sexual intercourse.* (He also found that histidine taken 4 g a day can help women regulate their periods.)

In males, excessive histidine was found to result in premature ejaculation, leading to frustration. *Where this is a problem Pfeiffer found that supplementation with 500 mg methionine, together with 500 mg magnesium and 50 mg vitamin B6 helped to normalize the excessive levels of histidine, and therefore the problem of premature ejaculation.* [1]

References
[1] Pfeiffer, C. *Mental and Elemental Nutrients,* Keats Publishers, New Canaan, 1981.

WOUND HEALING

Among the nutrient aids to wound healing are zinc, vitamins C and E and the amino acid arginine.

In an animal study involving rats a one per cent dietary supplement of arginine improved wound healing. Weight loss after the wound was reduced, the healing process was accelerated and the thymus gland, which is important in the body's defence (immune) function, increased in size. (Arginine is a stimulator of growth hormone from the pituitary and this is considered the means whereby it enhances wound healing.) The researchers state in conclusion, 'We suggest that supplemental arginine may provide safe nutritional means to improve wound healing and thymic function in injured and stressed humans.'[1]

References
[1] Barbul, A. et al. *Wound healing and thymotrophic effects of arginine,* American Journal of Clinical Nutrition, 37(5): 786, 1983.

5 CAUTIONS, COMBINATIONS AND DOSAGES

Because a nutrient, or anything else for that matter, is good for you in certain circumstances, at a particular dosage, it does not mean that you will always need it, or that more than that dosage will be even better for you.

Amino acids are no exception to this basic therapeutic rule.

As indicated in the main section of the book, in which we have looked at many of the therapeutic studies which prove the potential of amino acids to be real and exciting, the dosages vary considerably from a few hundred milligrams in some cases to several grams many times daily. It is suggested that the guidelines in that section and those listed below be followed, as long as there are no contraindications (also discussed below).

Caution

Phenylalanine (eg DLPA), tyrosine and tryptophan should never be taken when drugs of the class of *monoamine oxidase (MAO) inhibitors* are being used, as this could prove dangerous.

Arginine and *ornithine* should not be used by *schizophrenics* unless under supervision and *arginine* is not advised for individuals with active *herpes infection. Ornithine may be employed instead of arginine in such cases.*

Cysteine should not be used by *diabetics*, especially when insulin is being used.

Cystine should not be used by people with a tendency towards *kidney or bladder stones,* and the use of *cysteine* should always be accompanied by three times the dosage of vitamin C to ensure that excess cystine is not produced. Always take *histidine* together with vitamin C.

Histidine should be used cautiously by anyone with a *schizophrenic* condition as some forms (histadelic) show an excess of its derivative histamine. *Manic depressives* should also avoid *histidine. Histidine* in dosages of 4 g daily and over can result in *onset of menstruation.* This can be used to control the timing of the menstrual flow.

Aspartic acid may result in flatulence.

Methionine use should always be together *with vitamin B6 to avoid excess buildup of homocysteine.* It is also advisable to *always take magnesium when using methionine.* Methionine has a 'rotten egg' smell and should be used in capsule form to avoid this.

Anyone with *high blood pressure* who is taking medication for this should be cautious with use of *phenylalanine.*

Pregnant women or those lactating should avoid use of amino acid supplementation unless under strict guidance. Any woman anticipating conception or already pregnant should avoid use of tryptophan or phenylalanine.

Tyrosine should be avoided by anyone with melanoma.

Unless specifically advised do not use 'D' forms of amino acids except in the form of pain relieving DLPA or DPA amino acids. The 'L' form is the way nature makes amino acids.

Use of individual amino acids can result in imbalances being produced among the other amino acids. This calls for a close monitoring of long term usage of any single amino acid on its own. There is no such danger when carefully constructed blends of amino acids are prescribed to meet the needs observed in amino acid profiles, or when the full complement of amino acids is taken in their free form. For these reasons use of single amino acids should be restricted in self medication situations to brief periods of real need, not exceeding a few weeks. If a condition requires more than this amount of time to assist it, then professional advice should be sought.

Use of all 20 amino acids is suggested (ideally together with appropriate nutrient factors such as minerals and vitamins) at a time separate from individual amino acid intake, to ensure that a supply of all additional, and possibly deficient, amino acids is made available to the body. It is sometimes suggested that one should take amino acids at mealtimes but it is generally better to take them away from mealtimes, 90 minutes either side of a meal. Sometimes, as in the case of the use of tryptophan as an appetite modifier, a small amount of carbohydrate assists in the uptake of the amino acid (a little sugar or a biscuit will do nicely).

Dosages

Arginine: Up to 8 g daily.

Histidine: Between 1 and 6 g daily with vitamin C.

Leucine: 10 g daily for Parkinsonism.

Lysine: 500 to 1500 mg daily in herpes cases, with a doubling of dosage when there is an active infection.

Methionine: 200 to 1000 mg daily with magnesium and vitamin B6.

Phenylalanine: 100 to 500 mg daily.

DLPA: 750 mg three times daily for three weeks, and then double this if no pain relief noted, for a further three weeks.

DPA: 400 mg three times daily for three weeks and then double dosage for a further three weeks, if no pain relief noted.

Proline: 500 to 1000 mg daily with vitamin C.

Threonine: 150 to 500 mg daily.

Tryptophan: 1 g before sleep (with magnesium and B6), 2 to 3 g for pain control and depression in divided doses. Maximum dose about 6 g daily, enhanced by carbohydrate snack at time of taking. Also enhanced by taking vitamin B3 (niacinamide) in ratio of two parts tryptophan to one part niacinamide.

Valine: 1 g daily together with phenylalanine, methionine and tryptophan. Ratio should be 3(P): 2(V): 2(M): 1(T) in weight reduction formulation, taken before meals.

Taurine: 100 to 1000 mg daily in divided doses for epilepsy, reducing to maintenance dose of 50 mg daily.

Carnitine: 1 to 3 g daily in divided doses.

Cysteine and Cystine: 1 g three times daily for a month, then twice daily, in chronic ill health, together with vitamin B6.

Glutathione: 1 to 3 g daily.

Alanine: 200 to 600 mg daily.

Tyrosine: 2 g three times daily for depression (for two weeks). Ideal intake is 100 mg per kilo of body weight per day.

Read the studies in Chapter 4 and note the variations in dosage used. Take advice if in any doubt at all as to dosage required.

RESOURCES

For amino acid profiles in which both serum (blood) and urine are tested (and this is by far the most accurate way of discovering just what is happening in the body to the various amino acids and their multiple derivatives) contact:

In the US:

Tyson Associates
1661 Lincoln Boulevard
Santa Monica
California 90404
(213) 452-7844
They will supply details of how this service is available via trans-atlantic carrier (one of the major airlines), who will refrigerate samples so that they arrive in a state fit for analysis.
   Cost is in the region of £100 each for the two tests.

In the UK:

	Urine amino acid tests:
Klaire Laboratories	Medabolics Ltd
126 Acomb Road	14 Mount Pleasant Road
Acomb	Tunbridge Wells
York Y02 4EY	Kent TN1 1QU
(0904) 793231	(0892) 42609

For supplies of pure free form amino acids contact:

Larkhall Laboratories   Nature's Best
225 Putney Bridge Road   PO Box 1
London SW15 2PY   Tunbridge Wells
(081) 874 1130   Kent TN2 3EQ
                                   (0892) 34143

Natural Flow Ltd.
Green Farm Nutrition Centre
Burwash Common
East Sussex TN19 7LX
(0435) 882482

Recommended Reading

Leon Chaitow, *Amino Acids in Therapy* (Thorsons, 1985)
Robert Erdmann and Meirion Jones, *The Amino Revolution* (Century, 1987)
Michael Weiner, *Maximum Immunity* (Gateway Books, 1987)
Arnold and Barry Fox, *DLPA* (Long Shadow Books, 1986)
Stephen Davies and Alan Stewart, *Nutritional Medicine* (Pan, 1987)
Melvyn Werbach, *Nutritional Influences on Illness* (Thorsons, 1989)
Brian and Roberta Morgan, *Brain Food* (Michael Joseph, 1986)
William Philpott and Dwight Kalita, *Brain Allergies* (Keats, 1980)
Jeffrey Bland, *Your Personal Health Programme* (Thorsons, 1983)
Harold Gelb, *Killing Pain Without Prescription* (Harper and Row, 1986)
E. Cheraskin, W. Ringsdorf and J. Clark, *Diet and Diseases* (Keats, 1968)
Leslie Kenton, *Ageless Ageing* (Century Arrow, 1986)
Roger Williams, *Nutrition Against Disease* (Bantam, 1981)
Leon Chaitow, *Candida Albicans: Could Yeast be Your Problem?* (Thorsons, 1986)
Leon Chaitow, *The Radiation Protection Plan* (Thorsons, 1988)
Leon Chaitow, *The Beat Fatigue Workbook* (Thorsons, 1988)

Contact the following organizations for assistance with specific problems.

Action Against Allergy, 43 The Downs, London SW20 8HG
(081-947-5082)

New Approaches to Cancer, Addington Park, Maidstone, Kent (0732–848336)

Alcoholics Anonymous, PO Box 514, 11 Redcliffe Cardens, London SW10 9BQ

Tranx Release, 14 Moorfield Square, Southfields, Northampton NN3 5BD (0604–250976)

Tranquillizer Recovery, 17 Peel Road, Wealdstone, Middx (081-427-2065)

MIND, 22 Harley Street, London W1N 2ED (071-637-0741)

Schizophrenia Association, Dryn Hyfrid, The Crescent, Bangor LL57 2AG (0248–354048)

Foresight (Association for Promotion of Preconceptual Care), The Old Vicarage, Church Lane, Witley, Godalming, Surrey GU8 5PN (042–879–4500)

British Migraine Association, 178a High Road, Byfleet, Weybridge, Surrey KT14 7ED (09323–52468)

Herpes Association, c/o Spare Rib, 27 Clerkenwell Close, London EC1 0AT (071-609 9061)

Hyperactive Children's Support Group, 71 Whyke Lane, Chichester, West Sussex PO19 2LD

Myalgic Encephalomyelitis Association, Stanford-Le-Hope, Essex SS17 8EX

M.E. Action Campaign, PO Box 1, Carnwarth, Lanark ML11 8NH

Premenstrual Tension Advisory Service, Box 268, Hove, East Sussex BN3' 1RW (0273–771366) (also gives advice on the menopause, contraception, and nutrition).

The Terrence Higgins Trust, 52–54 Gray's Inn Road, London WC1. (071-831 0330 or 071-242 1010 (helpline)).

For practitioners who utilize nutritional medicine contact:

British Naturopathic and Osteopathic Association, 6 Netherhall Gardens, London NW3 5RR (01-435-8728)

British Society of Allergy and Environmental Medicine, Acorns, Romsey Road, Cadnam, Southampton SO4 2NN

INDEX